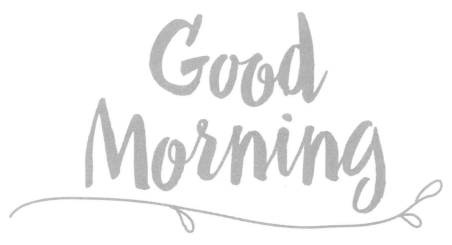

Good Morning

GOURMET BREAKFAST RECIPES

ANJA FORSNOR

PHOTOGRAPHY: CHARLOTTE GAWELL

h.f.ullmann

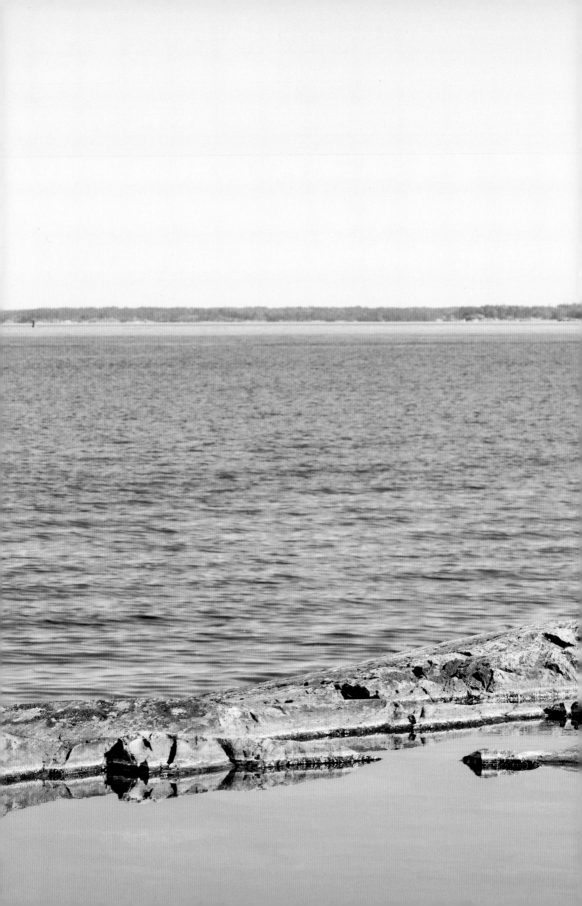

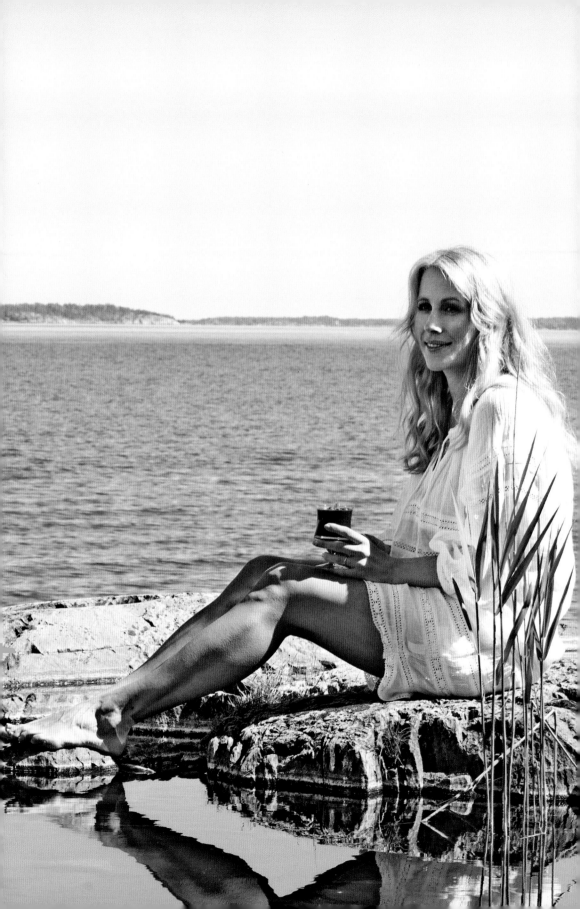

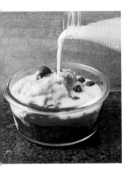
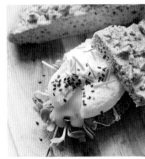
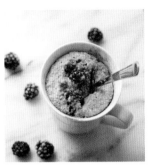
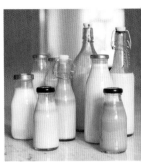

Table of Contents

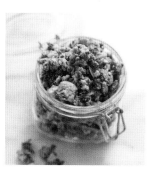 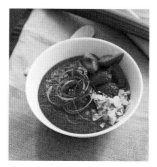 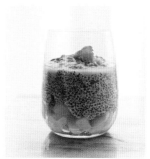 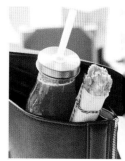

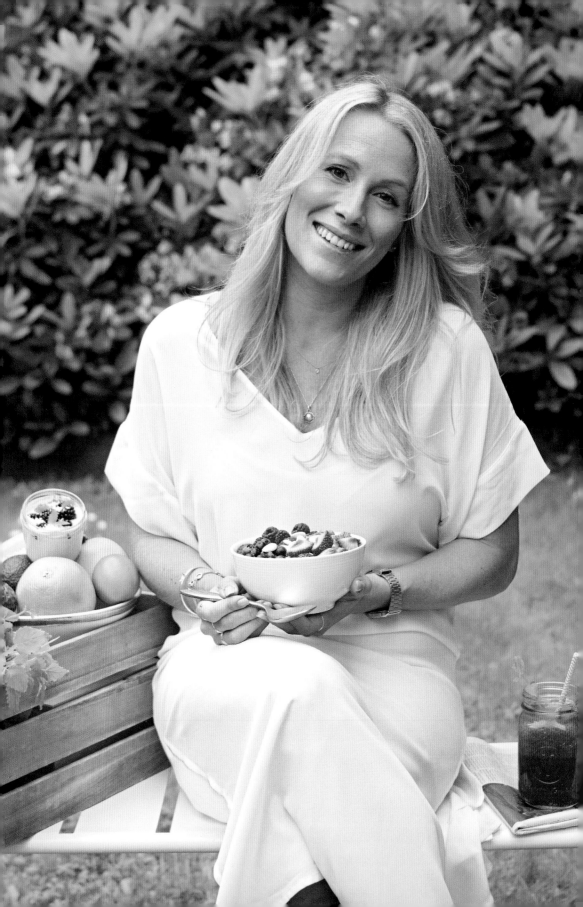

FOREWORD

YOU CAN ALMOST DIVIDE people into two groups —those who like to eat breakfast and those who do not. I belong to the former group and have been a breakfast person as long as I can remember. I am quite happy to set my alarm clock a bit earlier than is really needed so that I can eat my breakfast in leisurely fashion. For me, breakfast is the best meal of the day, and I could eat it several times over.

A European breakfast has long consisted of tea or coffee; bread served with meat, cheese, or preserves; and some yogurt. In Italy, you will be served a cup of black coffee and a sweet pastry, and in France a white coffee with a croissant. A British breakfast is more substantial and may include sausage, bacon, mushrooms, baked beans, scrambled egg, and toast with marmalade, and in the United States you will be offered pancakes with maple syrup.

Although we are influenced by flavors and spices from across the world, breakfast seems to be the one meal many of us find it difficult to make changes to, to the extent that we often take our breakfast habits with us when we are away from home or on holiday abroad. For some, breakfast is almost sacrosanct, and we will happily eat the same thing every morning, all year round.

So why do we hold on to our classic breakfast dishes with such tenacity? We have been eating porridge, bread with cheese, and yogurt since we were children, and yet never seem to tire of them. Perhaps it is because time is short in the mornings and we need something that is quick and simple and does not require too much thought. Or maybe it is about security—we just want something familiar with no frills.

Previously, like many other people, I ate the same thing for breakfast day in and day out. After years starting each day with porridge and apple purée, I acquired a blender and replaced my trusty porridge with smoothies. All of a sudden, a new world of alternative breakfasts opened up to me. Every day I blended fruit, vegetables, berries, and nuts into new favorites, and the combinations seemed endless.

As a nutrition advisor, I know that there are many benefits to eating breakfast, even though many people skip this first meal of the day. I am convinced that most of us do feel better for having something to eat in the morning. You simply need to establish a morning routine and good habits that work for your current lifestyle and for the longer term.

If you are looking for new ideas to inspire you in the kitchen in the morning, this book is for you. It contains tips for healthy, nutritious, tasty breakfasts that also work as between-meal snacks, pre-workout boosters, or evening nibbles. All the recipes are completely vegetarian as well as gluten-free and dairy-free, but you can of course use ordinary milk instead of nut milk if you prefer. My breakfast recipes aim to inspire you to make a greener start to your day that is simple, healthy, and absolutely delicious, with a message that is less "do not" and "must" and more about what is good for body and soul.

BEFORE YOU START

In this book I use alternatives to milk and wheat so that the recipes are suitable for as many people as possible irrespective of allergies or intolerances. If you have a nut allergy, many recipes work just as well if you replace the nuts with seeds.

Some of the ingredients may be unfamiliar, so I have given a brief description below. You will be able to find most of them in well-stocked food stores, in stores selling organic goods, or in health food stores, as well as online.

Ingredients

PSYLLIUM HUSK
Psyllium husk is a gluten-free fiber supplement made from the crushed husks of the psyllium seed. The fibers swell in contact with liquid and bind doughs together. I often use psyllium husk in my recipes as it has the same properties as wheat flour and gluten. You will find it in well-stocked food stores.

HAZELNUT FLOUR
Hazelnut flour is flour made from ground hazelnuts. It has a slightly nuttier flavor than almond flour and makes great-tasting bread. You will find hazelnut flour in the flour section of well-stocked food stores, but it is also easy to make yourself by grinding hazelnuts in a food processor.

PEANUT BUTTER
When not making my own peanut butter, I always buy organic peanut butter made from nothing but roasted peanuts and a little sea salt. Some brands contain large amounts of sugar, which I think is unnecessary, so I would advise you always to read the list of contents.

COCOA AND RAW CACAO POWDER
The production of cocoa involves such high temperatures that most of the nutrients are lost. Raw cacao is roasted at a lower temperature, so all the nutrients are retained. Raw cacao contains more antioxidants than any other food and also good fats, protein, iron, and magnesium.

Raw cacao is a little lighter in color, but the taste is largely the same. You can use ordinary cocoa instead of raw cacao in any of the recipes.

COCONUT FLOUR
Coconut flour is made by grinding coconut flesh into a fine flour. It has a sweet coconut flavor and works well in items such as muffins and cakes. You will find coconut flour in the flour section of well-stocked food stores. If you cannot find it in the stores, you can buy it online.

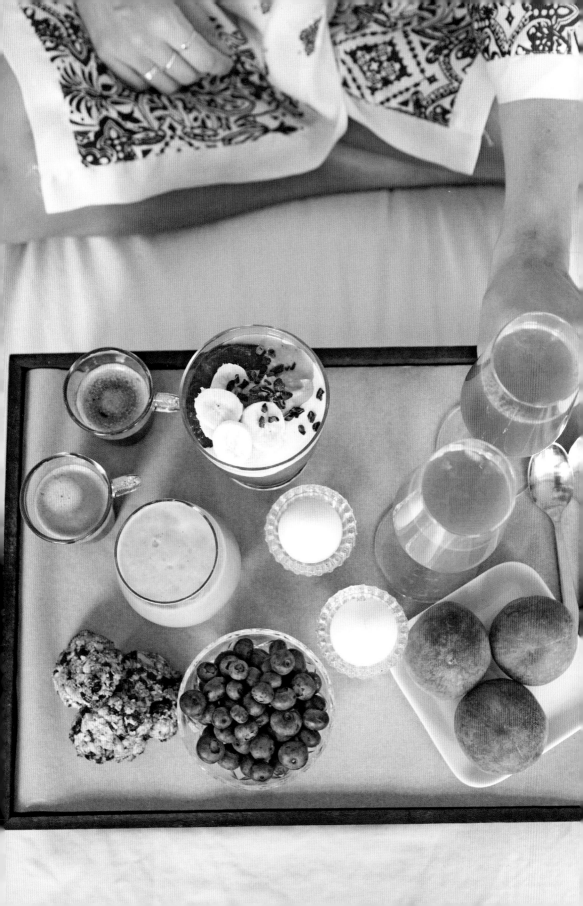

COCONUT OIL

I use organic, cold-pressed coconut oil for all types of food preparation, frying, and baking. Coconut oil is a healthy option because it is heat-resistant and is not altered by high temperatures. Cold-pressed means that during the production process it is never heated above 110 °F / 45 °C, so that it has the highest possible density of nutrients.

Coconut oil looks like a white paste; it will not melt below 75 °F / 25 °C. When using melted coconut oil in a recipe, I simply heat up a little oil in a few seconds either in the microwave or on the stovetop.

You will find cold-pressed coconut oil amongst the oils and vinegars in most food stores, or in your health food store. Cold-pressed coconut oil should not be confused with the fully hydrogenated, refined coconut fat that is sold alongside butters and margarines. It has none of the health benefits of cold-pressed oil. There are also odorless and flavorless versions of coconut oil for anyone who does not like coconut.

ALMOND FLOUR

Almond flour is a fine flour consisting of ground almonds. It contains a good deal of fat from the almonds and is great for slightly sweeter baked items such as muffins, scones, and bread. You will find it in the flour section of well-stocked food stores, or you can easily make it yourself by grinding almonds in a food processor.

ALMOND MILK

If you buy almond milk in the stores, you will usually have a number of different varieties to choose from, either sweetened or unsweetened. The sweetened variety usually contains large amounts of unnecessary sugar. I prefer the unsweetened version and then add natural sweetness in the form of dates, or other fruit, or honey.

I like to make my own almond milk, and for most bread and cake recipes I use it without any sweetener at all as I prefer the taste that way.

NUT BUTTER

I love nut butter in various forms, and use it a lot as a spread or as a flavoring for smoothies, bars, and cakes. It is very easy to make your own nut or almond butter—all you need is nuts, a little patience, and a really good food processor. See the recipe on page 128.

RICE MILK

Rice milk is made from water, rice, sunflower oil, and some sea salt. I like to use rice milk in smoothies, as the rice gives them a natural sweetness. My preference is for organic rice milk with added calcium; it is available in most well-stocked food stores.

VANILLA POWDER

Vanilla powder is made from vanilla pods that are ground into a fine powder. It has a strong vanilla flavor and is good for flavoring smoothies and cakes. In contrast to vanilla sugar, vanilla powder has no added sugar.

Kitchen equipment

FOOD PROCESSORS

I mainly use my food processor to make bread, raw food balls, and nut butter. Nuts and dried fruit can easily get stuck in a blender, so a food processor is perfect for these.

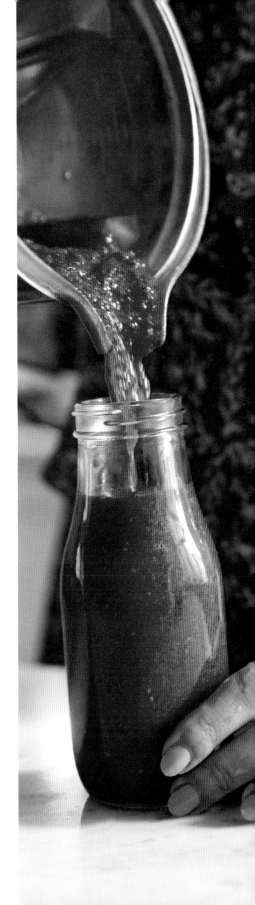

BLENDERS

I use my big blender every day for smoothies, fruit soups, and batters. My tip would be to invest in a blender that is powerful enough to blend ice, frozen berries, and frozen fruit. Remember that you must always add liquid to a blender so that your ingredients do not stick.

NUT MILK BAGS

If you want to make your own nut milk, I would suggest you invest in a nut milk bag. This is a nylon bag used to strain nut milk. Bags are easy to clean and can be reused time after time. You can also use them to strain juice if you do not have a juice extractor.

Nut milk bags are available online or you can buy them in well-stocked health food stores.

JUICE EXTRACTORS

A juice extractor is perfect for making juice from harder vegetables such as carrots, fennel, broccoli, or beets.

STICK BLENDERS

A stick blender is great for blending lighter items such as iced latte, banana ice cream, or pancake batter.

OVEN

All the temperatures given in the book are for a convection oven. For an ordinary oven, increase the temperature by 35 °F / 20 °C.

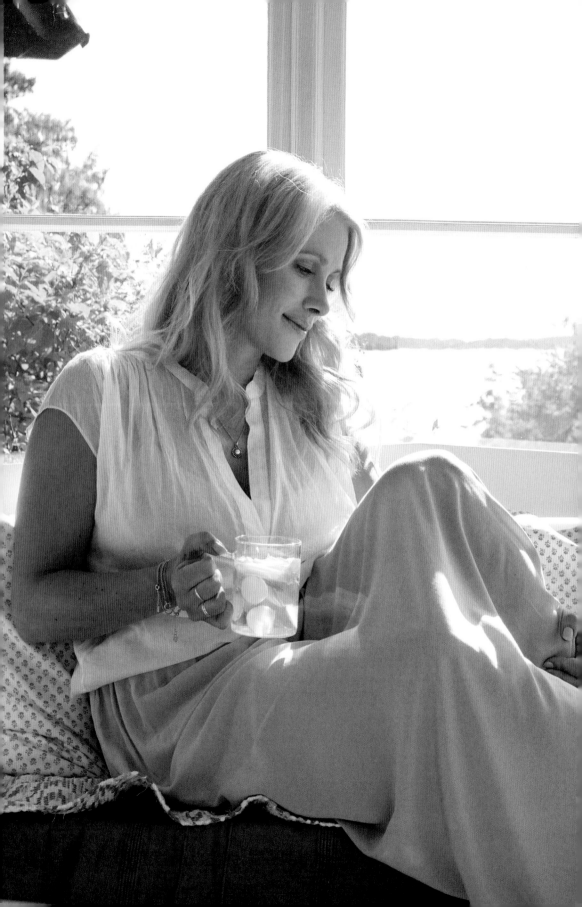

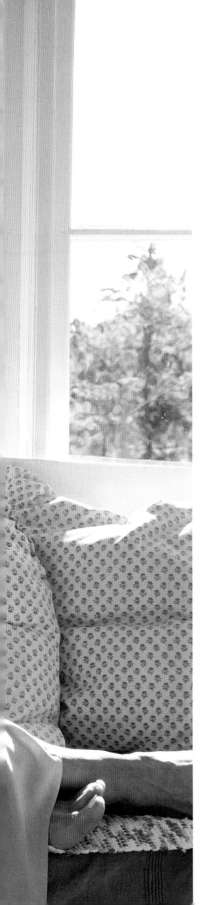

A great start to the day

BREAKFAST IS CONSIDERED to be the most important meal of the day, and I completely agree. It should kick-start your metabolism and fill your body with energy. Breakfast in the morning also raises your metabolic rate first thing after it has slowed down during the night. Whether you have a leisurely breakfast in bed at the weekend or on the jetty on a sunny summer's morning, or take something with you as you rush off to work, it provides a good start to the day.

I often sneak out of bed a bit earlier than my partner so that I can wake him up when breakfast is ready. I love that quiet time in the morning when I am busying myself in the kitchen and slowly getting myself ready for a new day. I always have a good supply of eggs, fruit, frozen berries, seeds, and nuts in the house so that I can easily throw together a breakfast without having to go to the stores.

I HAVE A NUMBER OF old favorites that I often fall back on, simply because they are the best way to wake up the body and they start my day off beautifully—these are breakfasts that make the body happy and keep hunger and blood sugar in balance until it is time for the next meal.

LEMON WATER WITH GINGER

Makes one glass

1¼ cups / 300 ml water
freshly-squeezed juice
   ½ organic lemon
1–2 cm / ½–¾ in. piece
   sliced fresh ginger
bunch of fresh mint
sliced lemon if wished

Lemon and ginger—two of my best friends. Make this your morning routine and your body will thank you for it. Not only is it delicious, it is also detoxifying and good for your immune system, digestion, and metabolism.

METHOD:

Bring the water to the boil and add the sliced ginger and the lemon juice. Top with a little fresh mint and allow to infuse for at least 10 minutes. It's a good idea to make a liter and store it in the fridge; it tastes just as good hot or cold.

Did you know?

Although lemon has a sour taste, it has an alkalizing effect on the body and combats damage from free radicals. It also curbs your sweet tooth! Ginger relieves nausea, has an anti-inflammatory effect, and also contains large amounts of antioxidants, which is helpful if you start to feel unwell.

Despite its strong taste, ginger has a calming effect on the stomach, reduces flatulence, and stimulates both the metabolism and digestion.

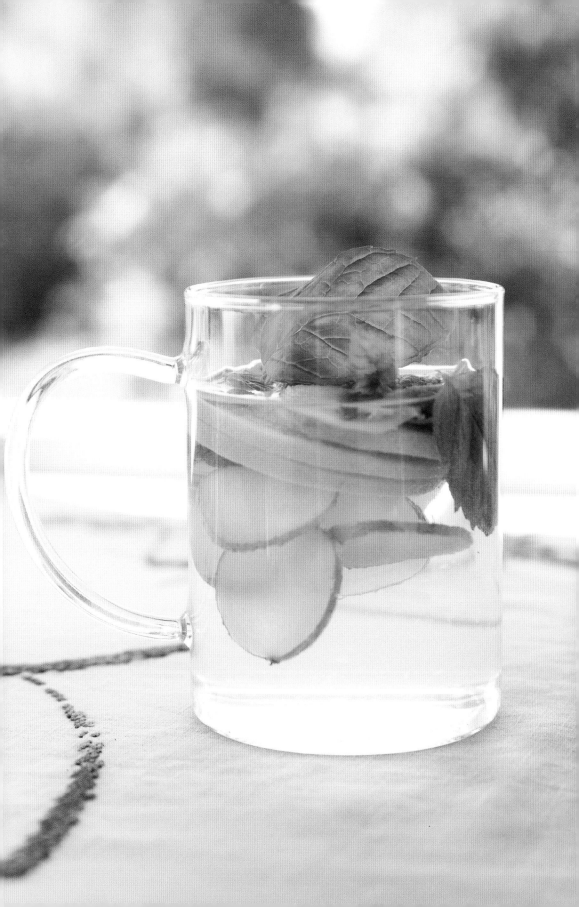

CRISPY BANANA PANCAKES

Makes one portion

1 ripe banana
1 egg
1 tbsp rolled oats
1 tsp psyllium husk
½ tsp ground cinnamon
½ tsp baking powder
salt

To serve:
berries
honey

What would a breakfast cookbook be without a recipe for the classic banana pancake? They're healthy, filling, and ridiculously tasty! Banana pancakes are perfect as a luxurious breakfast or snack, and popular with children and adults alike.

METHOD:
Blend all the ingredients using a stick blender. Allow to stand for five minutes so that the batter swells a little. Fry the pancakes in coconut oil over a medium heat. Serve with berries and drizzle over a little honey.

Tip

The base of these banana pancakes is equal quantities of eggs and bananas. I also like to mix in some baking powder, psyllium husk, and rolled oats to make them extra fluffy. The riper the bananas, the sweeter the pancakes.

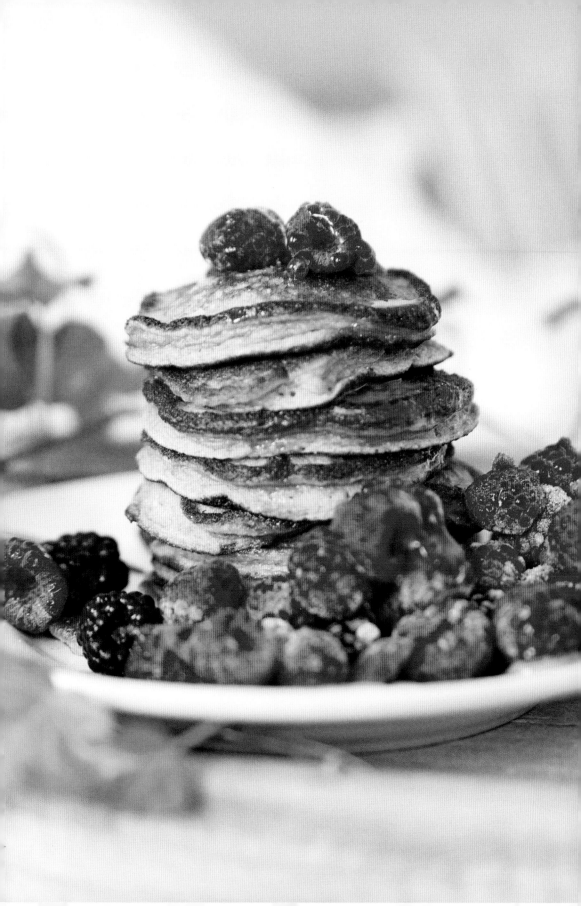

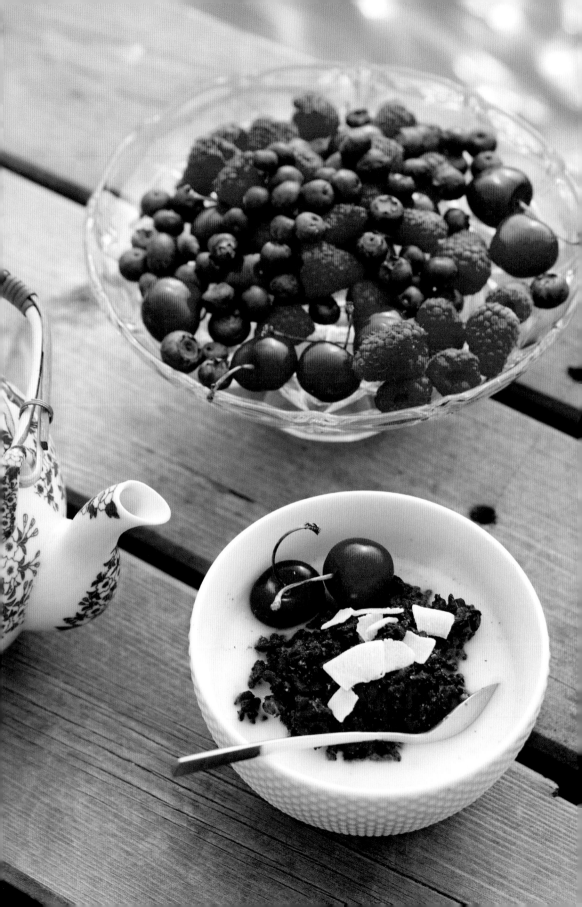

BLACK RICE PORRIDGE WITH CHERRIES

Not only is this rice porridge a feast for the eyes, it is really yummy too. Cooking the black rice in coconut milk makes the porridge sweet and filling. The black rice contains large amounts of healthy dietary fiber, antioxidants, protein, vitamins, and minerals—a real boost to your health!

METHOD:

Boil up the rice in seven tablespoons, or 100 ml, of water and 3½ tablespoons, or 50 ml, of coconut milk (i.e. do not use all the milk at once!) and allow to simmer on a low heat until all the liquid has been absorbed. Add the rest of the coconut milk and let the rice cook gently for about 30 minutes.

Stir in the honey and serve with toasted coconut, fresh cherries, and cold milk.

Makes one portion

3 oz / 85 g black rice
7 tbsp / 100 ml water
⅔ cup / 150 ml
    coconut milk
½ tbsp honey

To serve:
toasted coconut
fresh cherries
milk of your choice

BAGELS WITH CINNAMON AND RAISINS

Makes four bagels

2½ oz / 75 g buckwheat flour
2 oz / 55 g almond flour
1 oz / 30 g coconut flour
2 tbsp psyllium husk
2 tsp baking powder
2 tsp ground cinnamon
1 tsp vanilla powder
pinch salt
2 eggs + 1 egg yolk, beaten until light and fluffy
generous ¾ cup / 200 ml unsweetened almond milk
1 tsp apple cider vinegar
2 tsp honey
1 egg white, whisked to stiff peaks
1 oz / 30 g raisins

I developed my love of bagels when I was living and studying in the USA, and these ones with cinnamon and raisins are my favorite. If you toast them, you get a wonderful aroma like freshly-baked cinnamon buns.

METHOD:

Heat the oven to 390 °F / 200 °C. First put all the dry ingredients except the raisins into a bowl and mix. Beat 2 eggs and 1 egg yolk in another bowl until light and fluffy and add the milk, cider vinegar, honey, and, lastly, the dry ingredients. Whisk the egg white to stiff peaks in a separate bowl and stir them into the mixture together with the raisins. The mixture will become quite sticky. Allow to rest for 5 minutes.

Cover a baking tray with parchment paper. If you do not have any bagel forms, you could use suitably sized egg cups. Spoon some mixture around the egg cup to make your bagel shape, and remove the egg cup before you put the tray in the oven.

Bake the bagels in the middle of the oven for 20–25 minutes until golden brown. Allow to cool before serving.

Any that are not eaten can be stored in the fridge or frozen.

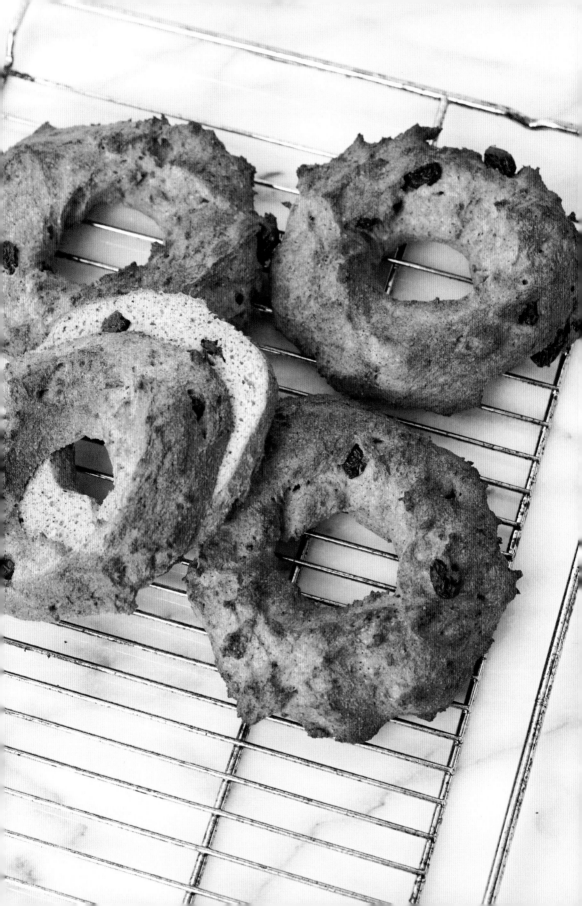

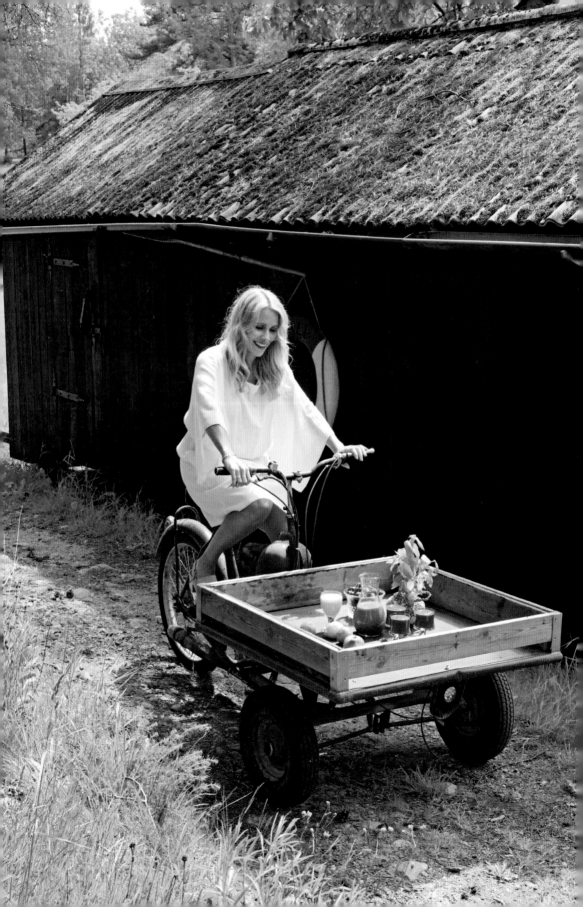

GOOD MORNING GREENS

A green start to the morning can never be wrong. This smoothie is really creamy and has a mild taste—perfect if green smoothies are new to you. You can also add half a teaspoonful of spirulina, chlorella, or wheatgrass if liked.

METHOD:
Blend all the ingredients in a blender, adding more coconut water if you prefer a more liquid smoothie. Pour into a glass and enjoy ice-cold. (See the picture overleaf).

Tip

I like to blend frozen peas into my green smoothies, as they give a lovely consistency and natural sweetness. Peas are also rich in protein, vitamin C, and dietary fiber, which is good for the digestion. I also like to add extras such as spirulina, chlorella, and wheatgrass to smoothies and juices.

Spirulina and chlorella are algae normally found in powder form; wheatgrass comes as both a juice and a powder. All three are rich in chlorophyll, protein, vitamins, and minerals, and are available from health food stores.

Makes one glass

generous ¾ cup / 200 ml coconut water
1½ oz / 40 g frozen spinach
½ banana
1¼ oz / 35 g frozen mango
¾ oz / 20 g frozen peas
juice ½ lime
¾ in. / 2 cm piece fresh ginger
ice

PINEAPPLE SMOOTHIE WITH ALOE VERA

Makes one glass

generous ¾ cup /
   200 ml almond milk
5 oz / 140 g frozen
   pineapple
1 ripe banana
juice ½ orange
2 tbsp aloe vera juice
ice

A fresh, energizing smoothie made from pineapple and aloe vera. Pineapple is rich in vitamin C, which strengthens the immune system and protects against free radicals. Pure aloe vera juice can have a bitter taste, but it is perfect in smoothies.

METHOD:
Blend all the ingredients in a blender, adding more almond milk if needed. Pour into a glass and enjoy ice-cold.

TANGY RASPBERRY SMOOTHIE

Makes one glass

generous ¾ cup /
   200 ml rice milk
3½ oz / 100 g frozen
   raspberries
½ ripe banana
pinch vanilla powder

A classic raspberry smoothie guarantees an energizing start to your day. This is a sweet-and-sour favorite, just packed with energy.

METHOD:
Blend all the ingredients in a blender, adding more rice milk if needed. Pour into a glass and enjoy ice-cold.

Did you know?

Raspberry is said to relieve menstrual pain in women, so be sure to fully indulge in raspberries when it is that time of the month. You will also be getting a dose of vitamins and minerals such as magnesium, calcium, phosphorus, and vitamin C.

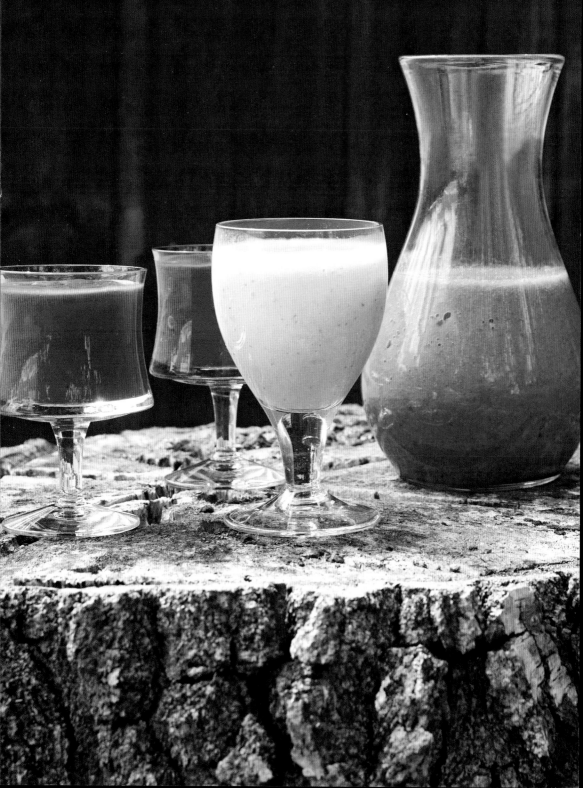

BANANA SCONES WITH BLUEBERRIES AND LEMON

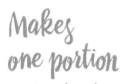

Makes one portion

2 oz / 55 g almond
  flour
1 tbsp coconut flour
1 tsp baking powder
1 ripe banana
1 egg
juice ½ lemon
1 tbsp blueberries

To garnish:
poppy seeds

These scones are absolutely delicious, and very easy to make. I often use banana in breakfast breads as it gives a good texture and natural sweetness. These are equally good eaten hot or cold.

METHOD:
Heat the oven to 390 °F / 200 °C. Mash the banana using a stick blender. Add the other ingredients and blend until you have a smooth mixture. Form the mixture into a large round circle (or two small ones) on a baking tray covered with parchment paper. Sprinkle with poppy seeds.

Bake in the oven for 10–12 minutes and serve with fresh blueberries.

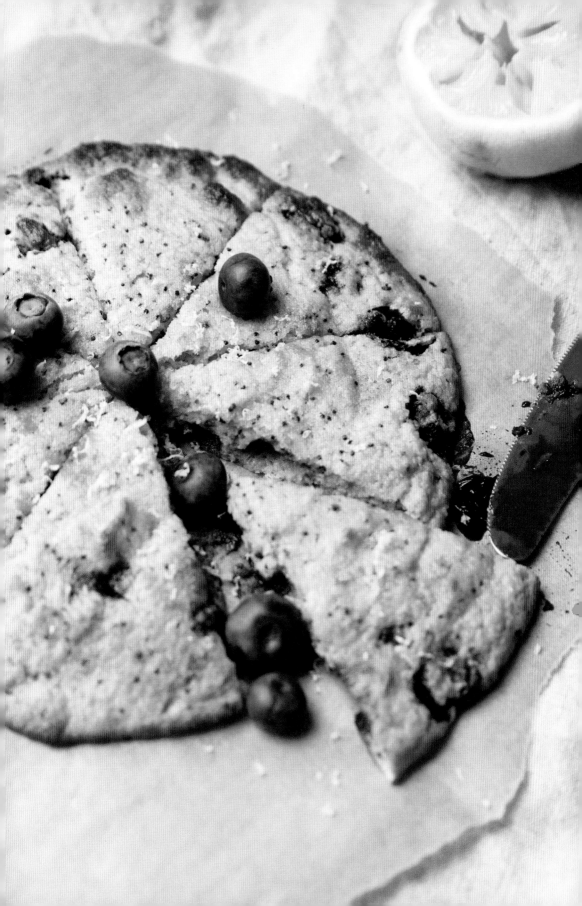

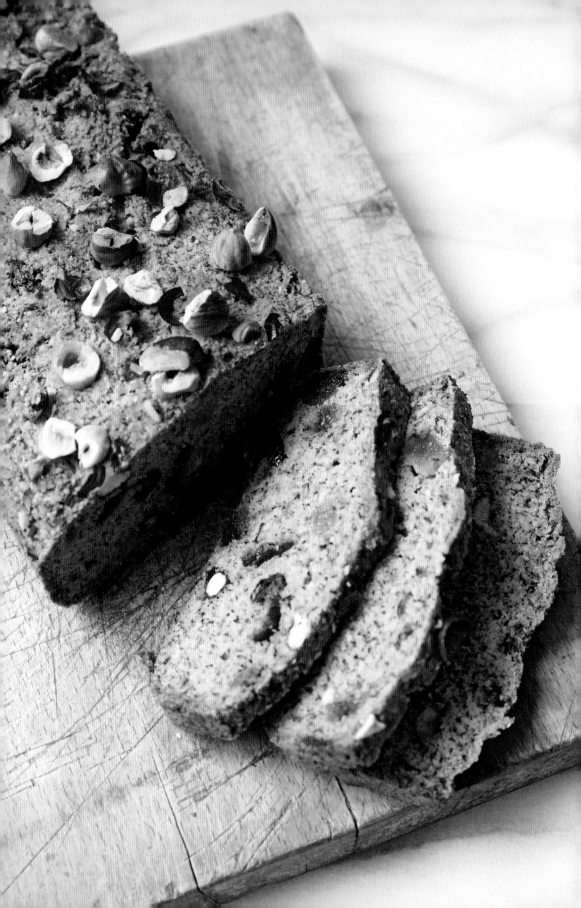

FRUIT-AND-NUT BREAD

A lovely, flavorsome bread with nuts and dried fruit. I have served this many times and it is always popular. It is perfect for storing in slices in the freezer.

METHOD:

Heat the oven to 390 °F / 200 °C. Mix all the dry ingredients, including the nuts, and add the raisins or cranberries and dried fruit. Stir in the egg, almond milk, and coconut oil. The mixture should be quite sticky and runny.

Line an oblong bread tin with parchment paper or grease it with a little coconut oil. Pour the mixture into the tin and top with some chopped nuts and fruit.

Bake in the center of the oven for about 50 minutes until the bread is a lovely golden brown color with a crispy crust. Allow to cool for a little while.

This bread is absolutely delicious with a piece of cheese and some jam, avocado, or nut butter (see recipe on page 128).

Stored in the fridge it will keep fresh and tasty for four or five days.

Tip

It is best to allow the bread to cool before slicing. Many gluten-free breads are best served cool, as the bread will often sag if you slice it straight away.

Makes one loaf

- 4½ oz / 125 g hazelnut flour
- 5 oz / 140 g almond flour
- 1 tbsp psyllium husk
- 1 oz / 25 g chopped nuts
- 2 tsp baking powder
- 1 tsp ground cinnamon
- ½ tsp ground cloves
- ½ tsp ground ginger
- pinch salt
- 1 oz / 30 g raisins or dried cranberries
- 2½ oz / 75 g dried fruit, e.g. dates, apricots, figs
- 2 eggs
- generous ¾ cup / 200 ml almond milk
- 2 tbsp melted, cold-pressed coconut oil

To garnish:
chopped nuts
dried fruit

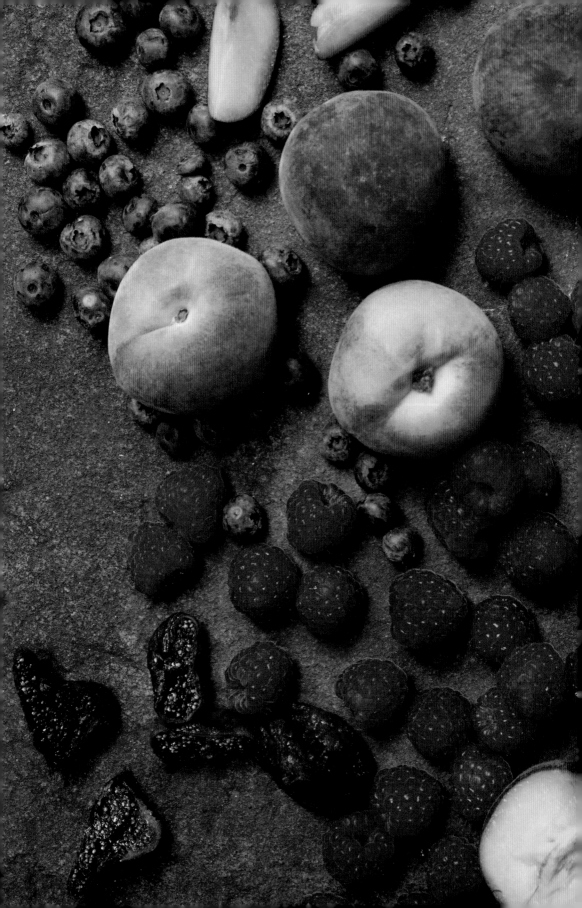

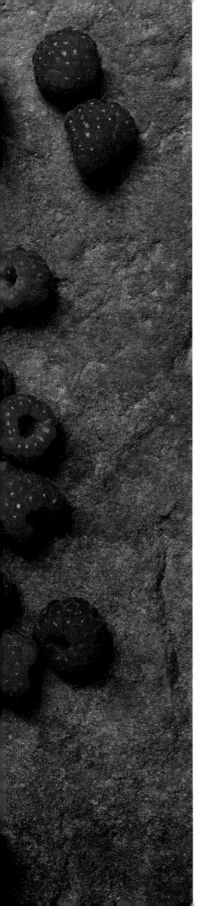

An energy boost

TOO LITTLE SLEEP? EARLY STARTS? Woken up by lively children? Some days you need an extra energy boost to get your body up and running. Have an invigorating shower and make a breakfast that will give you an energizing start to the day.

Avoid the traps of sugar and fast carbohydrates that will send your blood sugar sky-high. They will give you some short-term energy but your blood sugar will then fall, making you even more tired than before. Try slow carbohydrates instead, such as buckwheat or quinoa, and get natural energy from nuts, fruits, and berries.

If you often feel tired and lethargic even when you have slept well, it may be a good idea to review your eating habits. Begin with breakfast, and get your day off to a flying start. Try replacing what you normally eat for breakfast with one of the alternatives in this chapter, and you will soon notice a difference.

ACAÍ BOWL WITH FRESH BERRIES

Makes one portion

3½ oz / 100 g frozen acaí berries or 1–2 tbsp acaí powder

3 oz / 90 g frozen berries, e.g. raspberries, blueberries

1 banana

1 tsp honey (optional)

To serve:
berries, seeds, nuts

Colorful acaí bowls are commonly eaten for breakfast or as a snack both in the USA and in Brazil. When I lived in San Diego, we often had an acaí bowl as an indulgent weekend breakfast. They are a wonderful mixture of smoothie and frozen yogurt, packed with energy from the acaí superberry, one of the healthiest berries in the world—they will keep you on the ball all day!

METHOD:

Remove the bag of acaí berries from the freezer a little ahead of time, so that the berries defrost for a minute or two. To achieve the right texture, they should still be frozen when you blend them. Blend the acaí berries, other berries, and banana with a stick blender and flavor with some honey. Serve with berries, seeds, and nuts.

Did you know?

Containing large amounts of antioxidants, dietary fiber, and essential fats, the dark purple acaí berry is universally acclaimed as the healthiest berry in the world. The acaí palm tree is found in Central and South America and can reach a height of 80 feet / 25 meters. This means it gets a lot of sunlight, and so the berry can contain up to six times as many antioxidants as blueberries. Acaí berries are available as an additive in powder form or in packages of frozen, mixed berries.

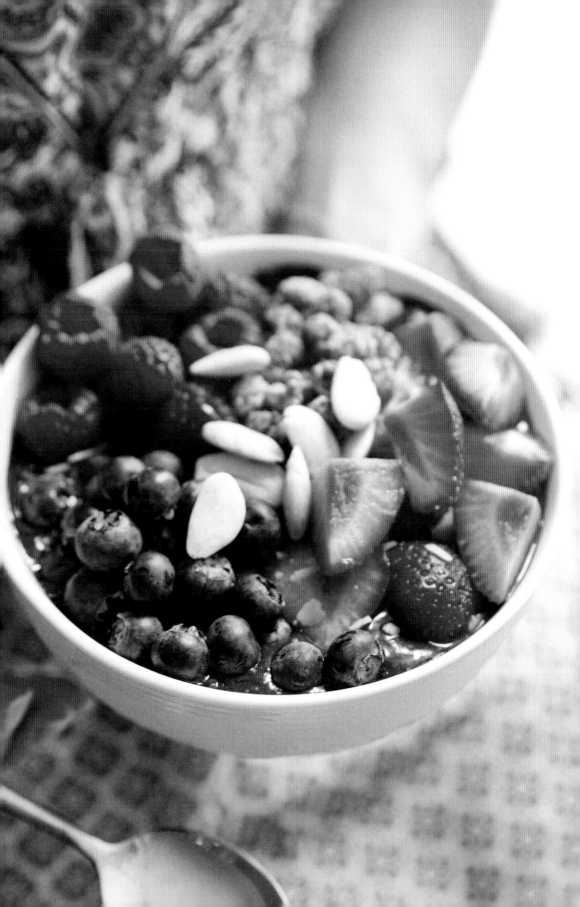

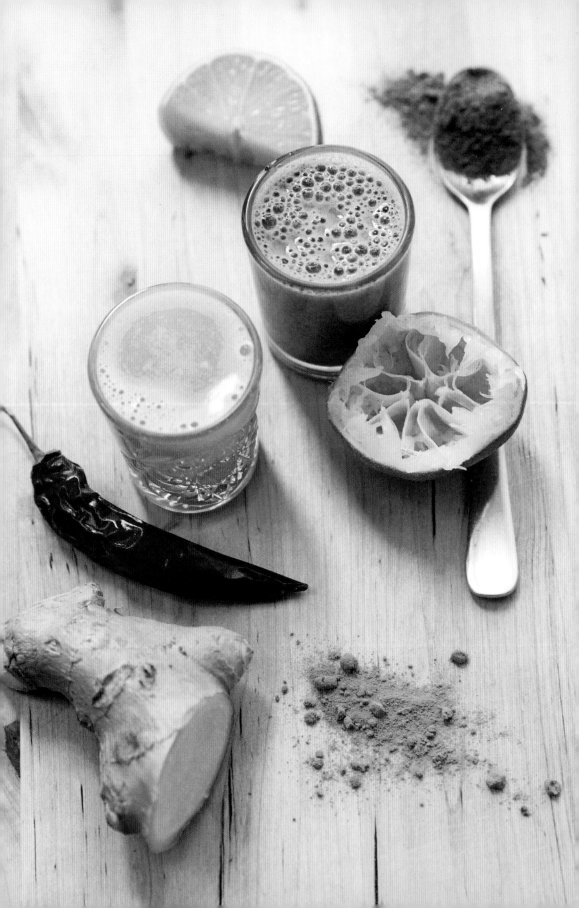

TURMERIC AND CAYENNE SHOT

Hot, spicy, and anti-inflammatory—few things are as invigorating as a powerful energy shot!

METHOD:
Blend all the ingredients using a stick blender or a jug blender, or shake them in a shaker. Pour into a glass and down in one go!

Did you know?

Turmeric is good for the digestion and the liver, and is full of antioxidants. It contains curcumin, which gives it its yellow color, and has been shown to have anti-inflammatory properties.

Makes one glass

7 tbsp / 100 ml freshly-pressed apple juice or water
1 tbsp dried turmeric
1 tbsp freshly-squeezed lemon juice
1 tsp ground cinnamon
¼ tsp cayenne pepper

SPINACH AND WHEATGRASS SHOT

This little glassful is packed with energy and will wake up your body in the best way possible.

METHOD:
Blend all the ingredients in a blender. Pour into a glass and down in one go! Cheers!

Did you know?

Wheatgrass powder is a green powder that contains, amongst other things, magnesium, chlorophyll, and zinc, which give an extra boost of energy. Alternatives to try include spirulina or chlorella.

Makes one glass

7 tbsp / 100 ml freshly-squeezed orange juice or water
5 fresh spinach leaves
1 tbsp freshly-squeezed lemon juice
1 tsp fresh ginger, grated
1 tsp wheatgrass powder

GRAPEFRUIT JUICE WITH APPLE

Makes two glasses

2 ruby/
  pink grapefruit
1 apple
ice

The perfect breakfast juice, both sweet and sour at the same time.

METHOD:
Peel the grapefruit and juice them together with the apple in a juice extractor. Serve immediately with a little ice, and enjoy.

Tip

If you don't have a juice extractor or juicer, you can make this juice just as easily in a blender. First peel and core the apple and chop it into small pieces. Blend the fruit with a little water and strain the resulting liquid using a strainer or a nut milk bag.

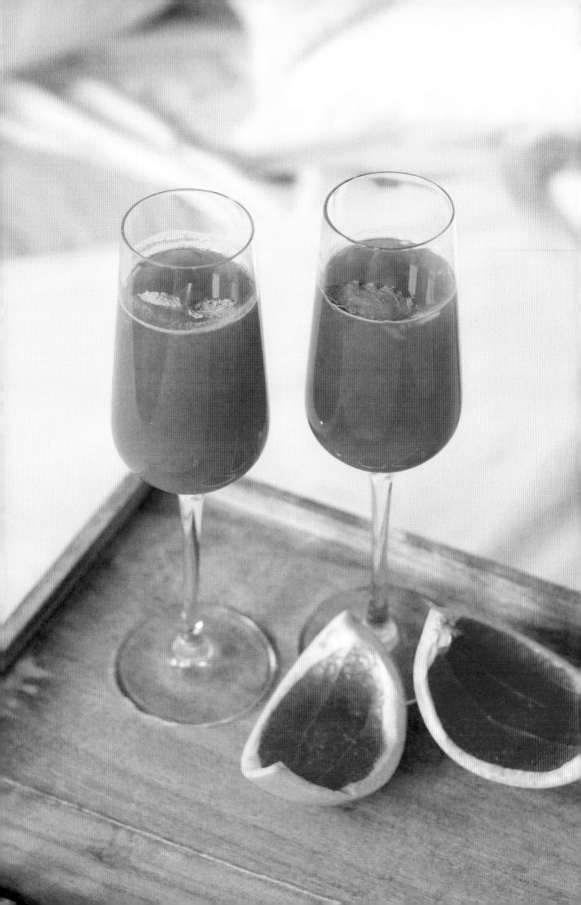

STRAWBERRY SOUP WITH COCONUT MILK AND MINT

Makes one portion

3½ oz / 100g fresh
  strawberries
3½ tbsp / 50 ml coconut
  milk
1 tbsp honey

To serve:
coconut milk
fresh mint
fresh strawberries

A delicious, creamy fruit soup made from fresh strawberries.

METHOD:
Blend the strawberries with the coconut milk and flavor with a little honey. Dribble a little whipped coconut milk over the soup and top with fresh strawberries and some mint.

Tip

I usually buy canned, organic coconut milk and store it in the pantry. It makes the perfect base for smoothies or porridge. Dilute with a little water if it is too thick or too fatty for your taste.

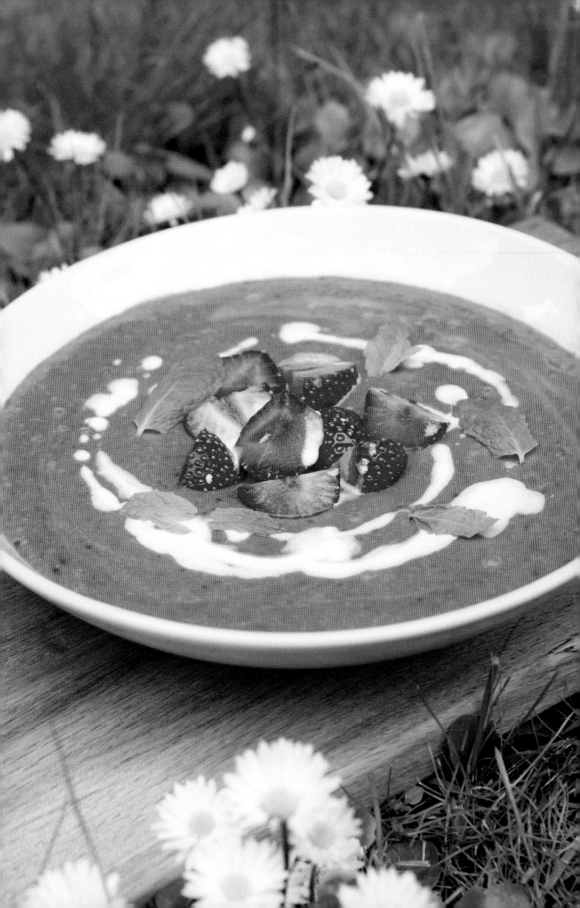

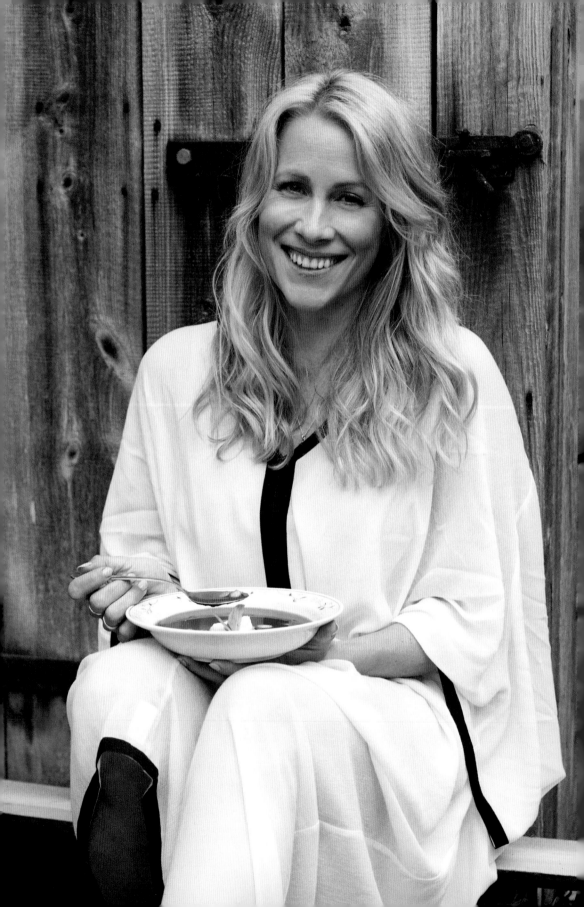

ROSEHIP SOUP WITH ORANGE AND HONEY-ROASTED ALMONDS

Few things take me back to my childhood as easily as rosehip soup. Rosehips are full of vitamin C, and the soup is equally good as a breakfast dish, a snack, or a hot drink to take on a picnic. It is really easy to make your own rosehip soup and so much healthier than the ready-made version you can buy in the stores. I like to make a big batch and keep it in the fridge for a few days.

METHOD:
Put the cold water into a saucepan and whisk the rosehip flour into it. Bring to the boil on a low heat and add the orange juice and honey.

Toast the almonds in a hot, dry frying pan and drizzle the honey over once the almonds have browned a little. Transfer them to a dish and allow to cool before serving so that they become really crunchy.

Top the soup with whipped coconut cream and roasted almonds.

Did you know?

Coconut cream can be found on the Asian food shelves in most food stores. It is creamier than ordinary coconut milk and can be used whipped or just as it is. Rosehip peel flour is made from dried rosehip peel, and is a slightly acidic flour that is rich in vitamin C. It can be used both for rosehip soup and in breads and cakes and is available in well-stocked food shops.

Makes one portion

generous ¾ cup / 200 ml water
½ oz / 15 g rosehip peel flour
juice ½ orange
1 tbsp honey

Honey-roasted almonds:
1¾ oz / 35 g whole almonds
1 tbsp honey

To serve:
3½ tbsp / 50 ml coconut cream

MATCHA ICED LATTE

Makes one glass

1 tsp matcha powder
1 tsp honey
3½ tbsp / 50 ml cold
   water
ice
generous ¾ cup /
   200 ml oat milk

I love this Japanese health drink, preferring it to coffee. In addition to its attractive green color, matcha is rich in antioxidants and amino acids, and has a calming effect.

METHOD:
Blend the matcha powder, honey, and cold water with a stick blender or a matcha whisk if you have one. Pour it into a glass with plenty of ice and top with foaming oat milk. For a warming latte, use hot milk and hot water instead.

Did you know?

This Japanese green tea has long been acclaimed for its health-giving properties, and is said to have a positive effect on blood count, improve cardiac health, and promote weight loss. Before matcha leaves are harvested, they are given protection from direct sunlight, which means that the leaves are packed with chlorophyll and nutrients. They also contain an amazing amount of antioxidants.

Matcha powder is sold in health food stores or well-stocked tea stores.

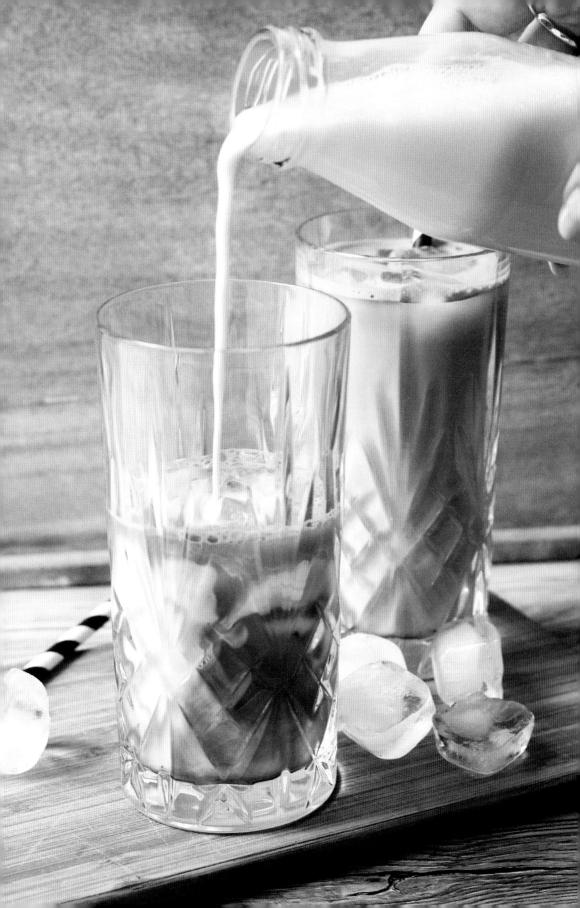

CASHEW YOGHURT WITH BLACKBERRIES

Makes one portion

4 oz / 120 g cashew nuts
generous ¾ cup /
    200 ml water
1 tsp vanilla powder

To serve:
fresh berries
shredded coconut
lemon balm

A yummy and filling alternative to ordinary yogurt, made from cashew nuts, water, and vanilla powder. The energy content of even a small portion of the nuts will keep hunger at bay for a long time. If you make a big batch, you can keep it in the fridge for three or four days, giving you breakfast for the whole week.

METHOD:
Soak the nuts for at least five hours, preferably overnight. Drain off the water and blend the nuts in a blender with seven tablespoons, or 100 ml, of water. Then add the remaining seven tablespoons, or 100 ml, of water or more until you have the desired consistency, and flavor with the vanilla powder.

Serve with fresh berries, shredded coconut, and lemon balm.

Tip

Vary the flavor of your cashew yogurt by blending frozen berries, banana, or a little cinnamon along with the nuts.

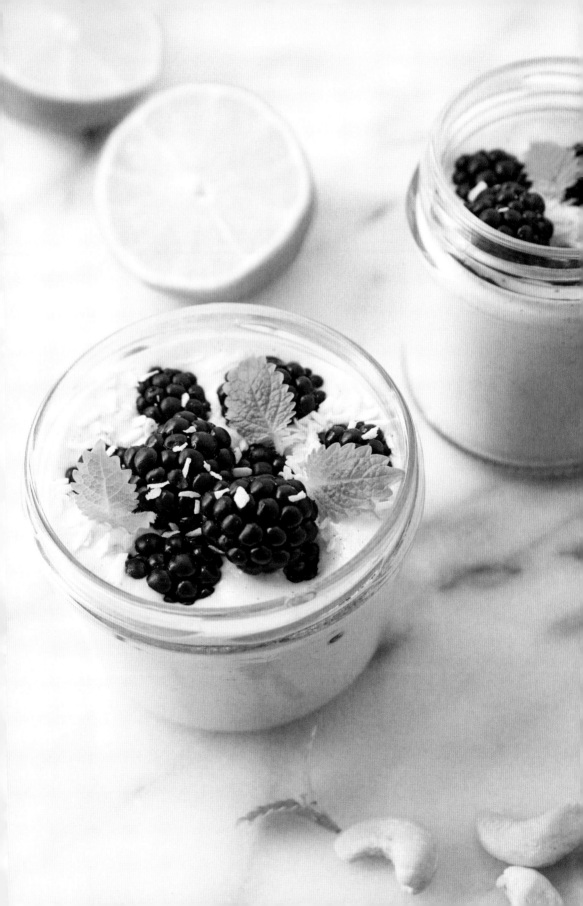

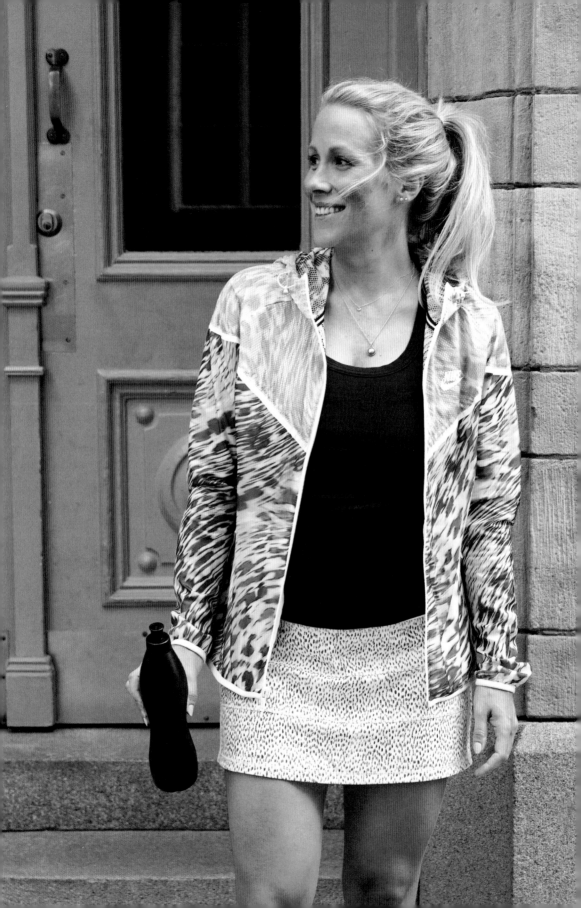

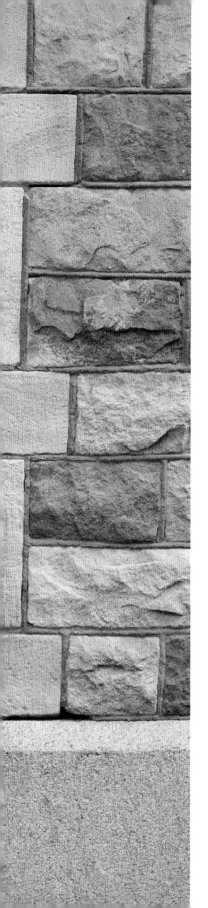

Breakfast and exercise

IT'S NO SECRET THAT WHAT YOU EAT has a major impact on your exercising—food is important for energy levels, muscle development, and recovery. When you work out in the morning, it can be a good idea to have breakfast in two stages, so that you eat something both before and after your session. If you find it hard to eat in the morning, try something light, such as eggs, nuts, or a smoothie, so that you get some energy intake and can get the most out of your workout—then eat a slightly bigger breakfast afterwards to help your body recover. Breakfast never tastes better than when eaten after a sweaty exercise session!

This chapter contains recipes that will help you run further, give you more stamina, and help you recover more quickly—they all work equally well as breakfast or as high-energy snacks.

CHIA FRESCA

Makes one glass

1 cup / 250 ml water
1 tbsp chia seeds
juice 1 lime
honey according
  to taste

Chia fresca is a crisp, refreshing drink full of omega-3, protein, vitamins, and minerals. It is known as nature's energy drink, and is said to improve physical performance. Perfect for drinking before a workout to give you an energy boost.

METHOD:
Put the water and chia seeds into a glass, allow the seeds to swell for a few minutes, and then stir. Add the lime juice and sweeten with honey to taste.

When I drink it first thing in the morning, I add a smaller amount of honey so that it is really refreshing.

Did you know?

The Tarahumara people of Mexico are known for their ability to run amazingly long distances without tiring. Their secret is said to be their habit of drinking chia fresca to help them recover and gather new strength. It is tempting, isn't it!

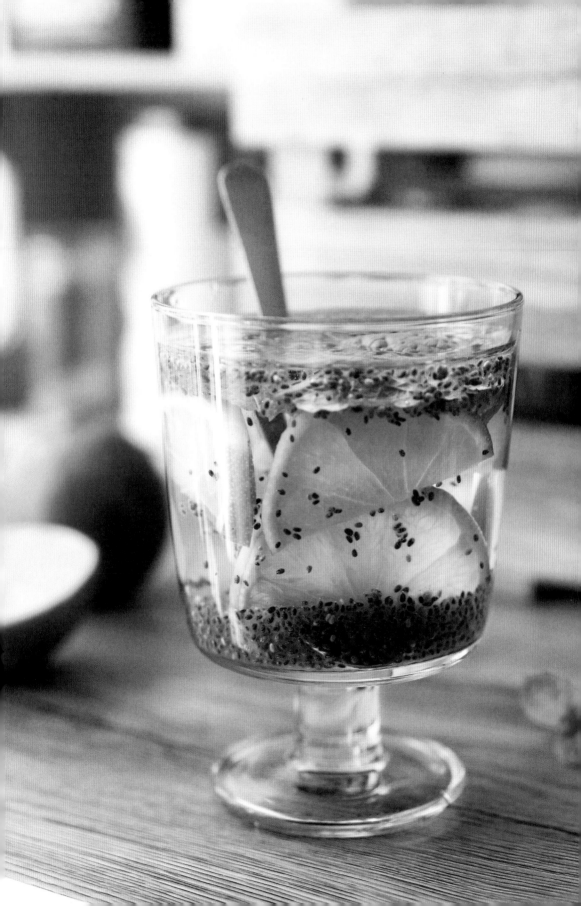

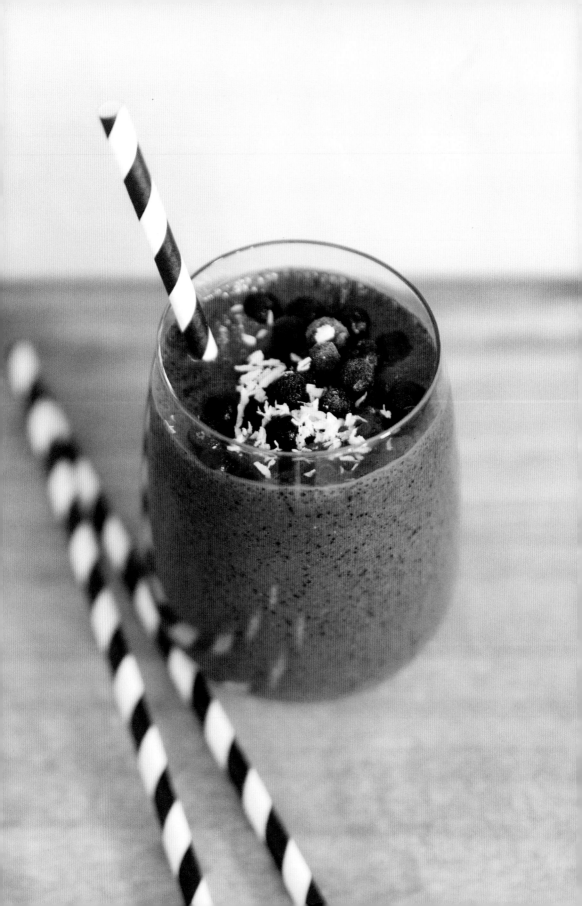

PROTEIN SMOOTHIE WITH OATS AND BLUEBERRIES

A delicious, protein-rich breakfast smoothie that will go down easily both before and after your workout. Blending an egg into the smoothie provides extra protein, which is good for helping muscles recover, and also makes it filling.

METHOD:
Blend all the ingredients in a blender, adding more oat milk if needed. Pour into a glass and enjoy ice-cold, preferably topped with blueberries and some coconut.

Tip

Oats are a fantastic food, containing both healthy fat and protein. They also contain whole grains, antioxidants, dietary fiber, vitamins, and minerals. I like blending oats into my smoothie; they make it slightly thicker, and the combination of oats, banana, and cinnamon makes for a real breakfast taste. If you don't want porridge for breakfast, this is the perfect alternative way to enjoy all the benefits of oats.

Makes one glass

generous ¾ cup / 200 ml oat milk
2 oz / 60 g frozen blueberries
1¼ oz / 35 g rolled oats
1 banana
1 egg
1 tsp cold-pressed coconut oil
½ tsp ground cinnamon
ice

Topping:
blueberries
shredded coconut

RAWGHURT WITH RASPBERRIES

Makes one portion

2½ oz / 75 g frozen
  raspberries
1 ripe avocado
½ frozen banana
3 tbsp pea protein
  or hemp protein
  (optional)

Topping:
seeds
dried berries

Rawghurt is a vegan yogurt that uses avocado as a base. It has a really creamy texture and can be flavored with different types of fruit, greens, and berries. A good way of getting energy in the form of beneficial fats.

METHOD:
If you can, take the berries from the freezer a few minutes in advance so that they do not stick in the blender. The easiest method is to blend all the ingredients using a stick blender. If you use an ordinary blender, you may need to add some liquid, for example almond milk or water.

Did you know?

Protein powder is a good way to boost your breakfast when you're exercising. I like to use vanilla-flavored whey protein isolate or a vegetable alternative such as pea protein or hemp protein.

Protein powder can be bought from health food stores or online outlets, as well as from stores specializing in food supplements for training and sports performance.

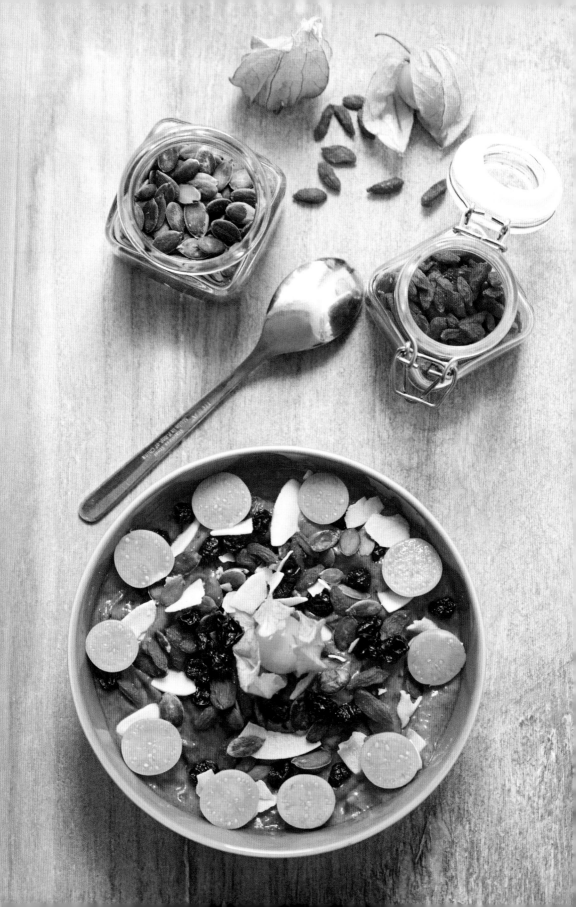

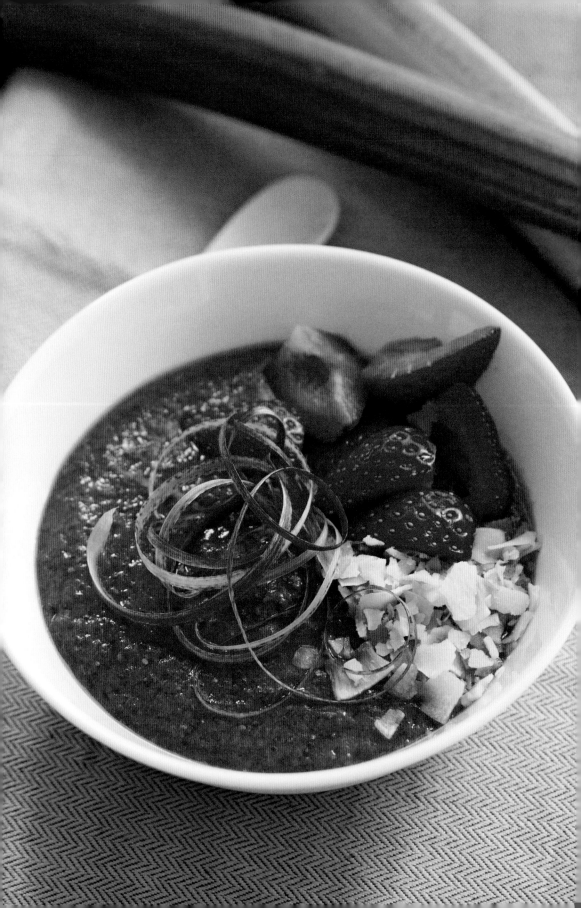

CHIA CREAM WITH RHUBARB AND STRAWBERRIES

A cross between porridge and fruit cream that's healthy and tasty. You can very easily prepare this before your workout to be enjoyed when you come home.

METHOD:
Slice the strawberries and rhubarb, put it all into a saucepan on the stovetop and bring to the boil. Blend with a stick blender and add the chia seeds. Flavor with honey and vanilla powder and allow to cool before serving. It's very easy to make a double portion of this and store it in the fridge.

Did you know?

Chia seeds are getting lots of attention as they are real nutritional bombs—they contain *eight times* as much omega-3 as salmon.

Makes one portion

3½ oz / 100 g strawberries
2 oz / 60 g rhubarb
3 tbsp chia seeds
2 tsp honey
pinch vanilla powder

REFRESHING WATERMELON SLUSH

Makes one glass

¾ lb / 340 g fresh
  watermelon, cubed
1 bunch fresh mint
ice

A slush made from watermelon is both healthy and thirst-quenching. Watermelon is a real health bomb and, according to studies, if eaten an hour before a training session it will stop you having sore muscles the following day. This is because watermelon is rich in an amino acid that helps blood vessels to relax and improves circulation. And that is a very good thing!

METHOD:
Blend the watermelon together with the mint and the ice. Because watermelon is largely water, no additional liquid is needed. Serve with ice and drink straight away.

Did you know?

Watermelon contains amino acids that the body converts into arginine, which has a positive impact on both the immune system and the heart. It also speeds up fat burning and helps the body build muscle. In addition, watermelon is 92% water, so it is an excellent way to get the water you need on a hot summer's day.

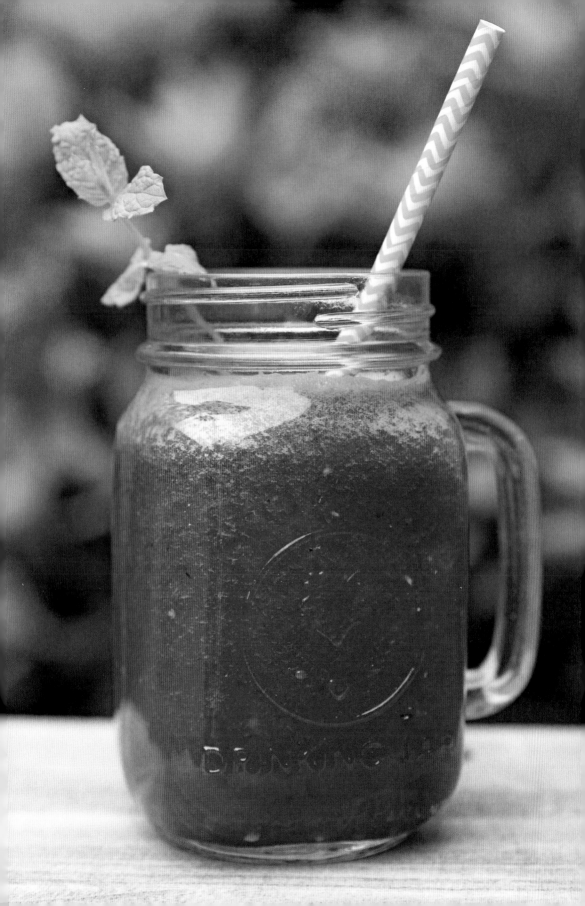

GREEN SMOOTHIE BOWL

Makes one portion

7 tbsp / 100 ml
  unsweetened almond
  milk
1 frozen banana
2½ oz / 70 g frozen
  mango
1¾ oz / 50 g frozen kale
½ avocado
2 tbsp freshly-squeezed
  lemon juice
1 tsp cold-pressed
  coconut oil
¾– 1¼ in. / 2–3 cm piece
  ginger
1 tsp flaxseeds
ice

Topping:
kiwi, banana, mango
seeds

I like to vary my smoothies with creamy smoothie bowls. By adding less liquid than you would normally add to a smoothie, you get a thicker version that can be eaten with a spoon. This favorite of mine is packed with green nourishment that is good for the body.

METHOD:
Blend all the ingredients into a smooth, creamy smoothie in a jug blender (a stick blender will not do the trick here). Top with kiwi, banana, mango, and plenty of seeds.

Did you know?

Kale is a real supervegetable! Rich in both calcium and omega-3, fresh or frozen kale is the perfect ingredient for your smoothie when you are exercising.

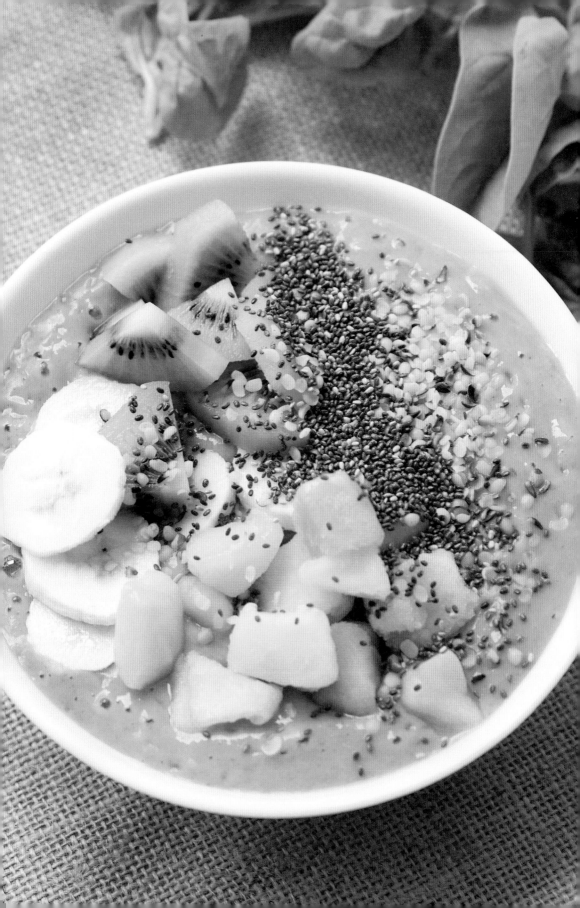

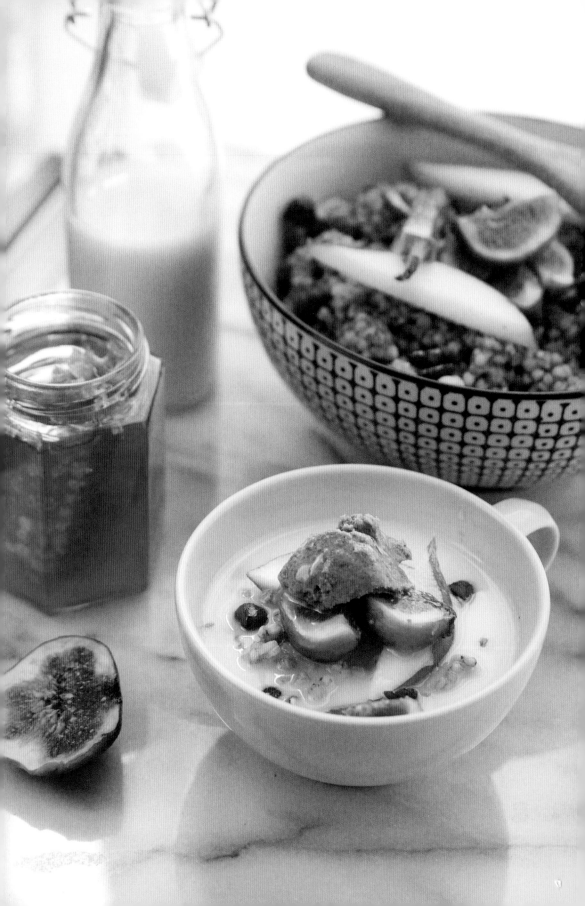

BUCKWHEAT PORRIDGE WITH FIG, PEAR, AND TAHINI

A tasty, gluten-free porridge made from buckwheat with the wonderful aroma of cinnamon. Tahini is a brilliant flavoring that goes perfectly with pears and fresh figs.

METHOD:
Cook the buckwheat according to the instructions on the packaging—about 15 minutes. Drain off any excess water and flavor with vanilla powder, cinnamon, and sea salt flakes.

Top the porridge with fresh figs, pear, hazelnuts, a dollop of tahini, a little honey, and some cold milk.

Did you know?

Buckwheat is not a grain but a plant that is extremely rich in minerals and good, slow carbohydrates that keep hunger at bay for a long time. Buckwheat is a little bit like rice and has little taste of its own, so you can flavor it in the way you prefer.

Makes one portion

3 oz / 80 g whole buckwheat (or 7 tbsp / 100 ml cooked)
pinch vanilla powder
pinch ground cinnamon
small pinch sea salt flakes

Topping:
fresh figs
pear
hazelnuts
tahini
honey
milk of your choice

WHOLE BUCKWHEAT WITH FRIED EGG

Makes one portion

3 oz / 80 g whole
   buckwheat (or 7 tbsp /
   100 ml cooked)
1 tsp olive oil
Small pinch paprika
salt and pepper
1 egg
1 spring onion

A substantial breakfast that I like to eat after my morning workout, when I do not fancy anything sweet. I often have cooked buckwheat in the fridge, so I can put this dish together in just a few minutes. Three ounces, or 80 g, of buckwheat is about seven tablespoons, or 100 ml, when cooked, which is exactly the amount needed in this recipe.

METHOD:
Cook the buckwheat according to the instructions on the packaging. Stir in a little olive oil and season as desired, perhaps with salt, pepper, and some paprika. Fry the egg, making sure the yolk remains creamy. Serve the buckwheat with the egg and chopped spring onion.

Did you know?

It is not by chance that eggs often feature in the context of breakfast. Eggs contain important vitamins and protein that keep hunger at bay longer so we don't feel the need to snack.

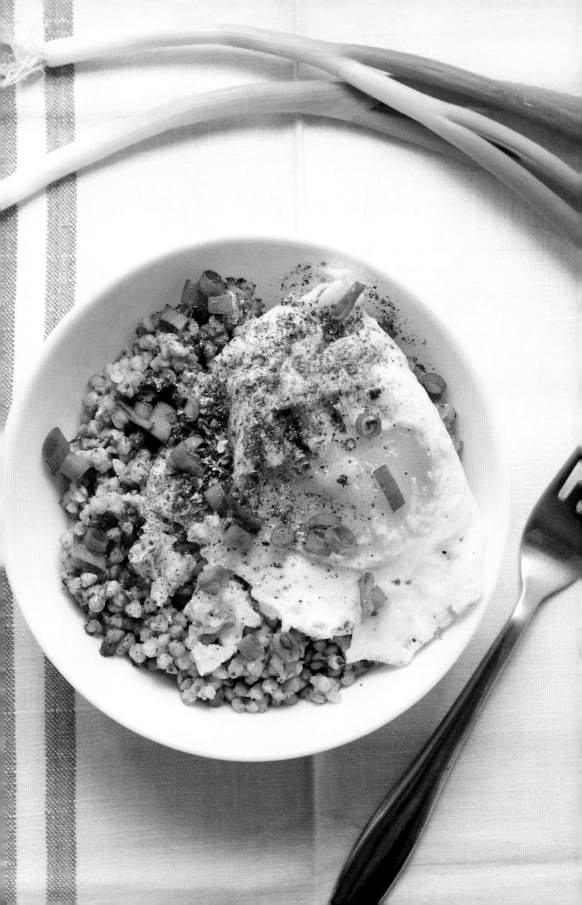

BEET SMOOTHIE WITH RAW CACAO

Makes one portion

generous ¾ cup /
  200 ml unsweetened
  almond milk
1¾ oz / 50 g frozen
  raspberries
juice ½ orange
1 cooked beet
1 tbsp raw cacao powder
1 tsp honey
½ tsp vanilla powder

I love beets and think they are particularly delicious in juices and smoothies. This is a real supersmoothie that will make your body rejoice!

METHOD:
Blend all the ingredients in a blender, adding more almond milk if needed. Pour into a glass and enjoy ice-cold.

Did you know?

Beets are a real superfood. In studies, they have been shown to improve both endurance and performance when exercising. The nitrates in the beets supply the muscles with more oxygen, making them the perfect food before your workout.

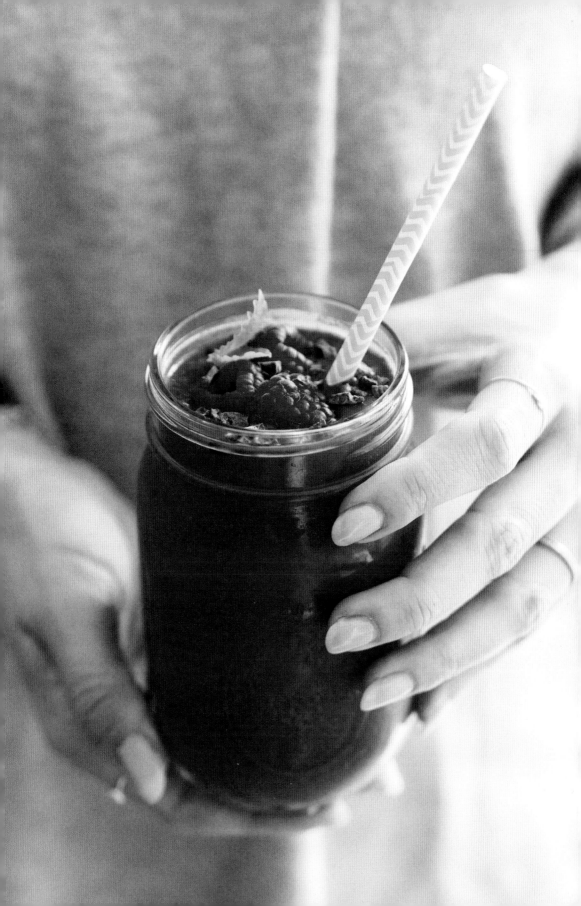

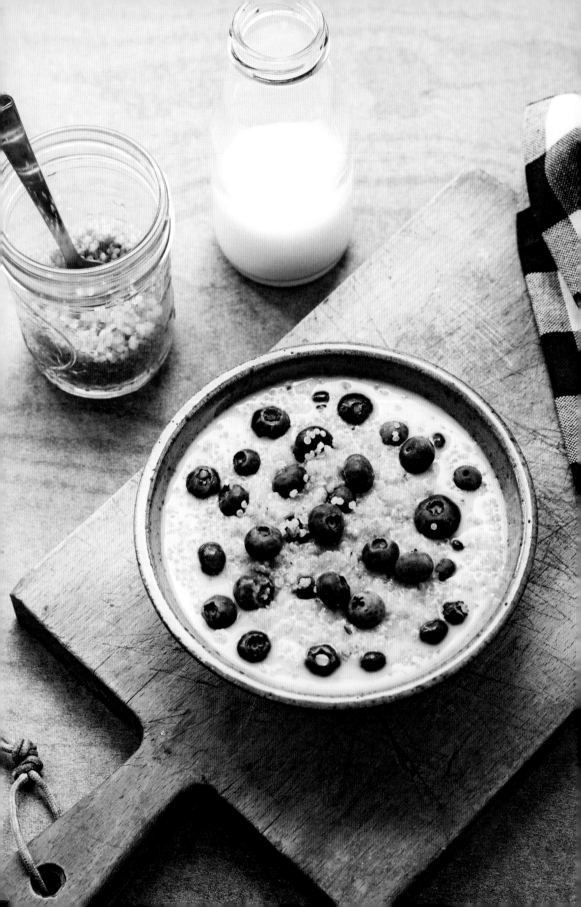

HOT QUINOA PORRIDGE

A delicious, energizing start to the day. Quinoa is a plant that is rich in protein, calcium, potassium, and iron. Blueberries contain vitamin C, dietary fiber, and antioxidants, and together they make a real superbreakfast. Cook a little extra quinoa so that you have breakfast ready-made for several days.

METHOD:
Boil the water, add the quinoa, and cook on a medium heat for 20 minutes. Stir the cinnamon into the quinoa and serve with fresh blueberries and rice milk. The porridge tastes just as good cold.

Makes one portion

generous ¾ cup /
   200 ml water
3 oz / 80 g quinoa (or
   2½ oz / 70 g cooked)
1 tsp ground cinnamon

To serve:
fresh blueberries
cold rice milk

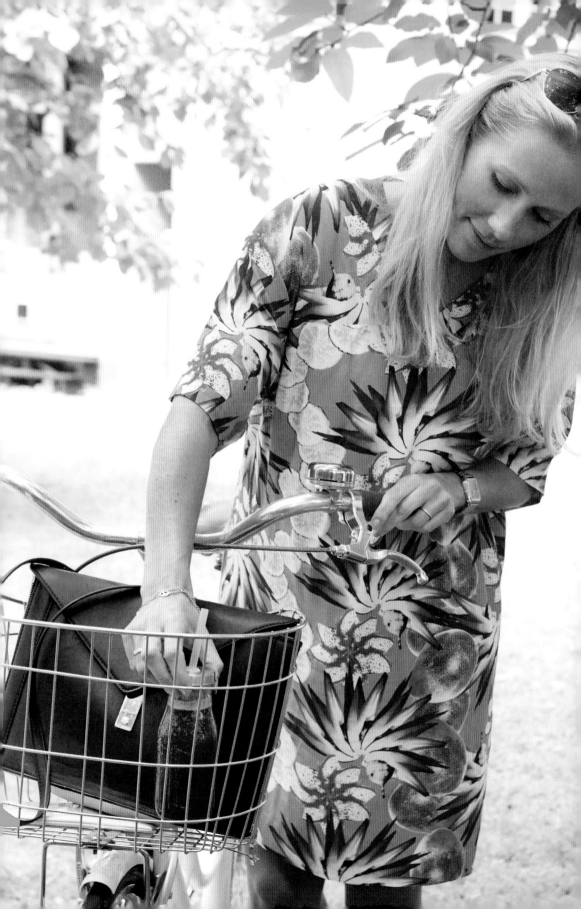

Breakfast when time is short

HOW DO YOU INCLUDE A HEALTHY, tasty breakfast in your schedule when you are in a hurry? Stressful mornings can spoil the day for even the cheeriest of us, and that makes regular breakfast habits even more important. Some days the time optimist in me takes over so I don't have as much time as I thought, and that calm breakfast moment I had been looking forward to is blown away. Rushing out of the house without eating anything does not work for me—it ruins my whole day and my mood takes a nosedive. But there is always something that you can throw together in a matter of moments; all that's needed is some imagination!

This chapter describes some speedy breakfasts that all take less than five minutes to prepare. I do think that you can always find at least a few minutes to spare, even when time is racing away.

If you are often short of time in the mornings, do not miss the recipes in the chapter after this, where you'll get tips for healthy breakfasts that are easy to prepare the night before.

CREAMY SCRAMBLED EGGS

Makes one portion

2 eggs
1 tbsp oat cream
½ tsp cold-pressed
  coconut oil
salt and pepper

Eggs must be the optimal food option when you are short of time. They are quick to prepare, rich in protein, satisfying, and also quite delicious. I make my scrambled eggs in a saucepan to ensure I get the perfect creamy consistency.

METHOD:
Heat the coconut oil in a saucepan. Whisk the eggs and oat cream with a fork and pour into the saucepan. Cook on a medium heat, stirring constantly, and season with salt and pepper. Serve with vegetables!

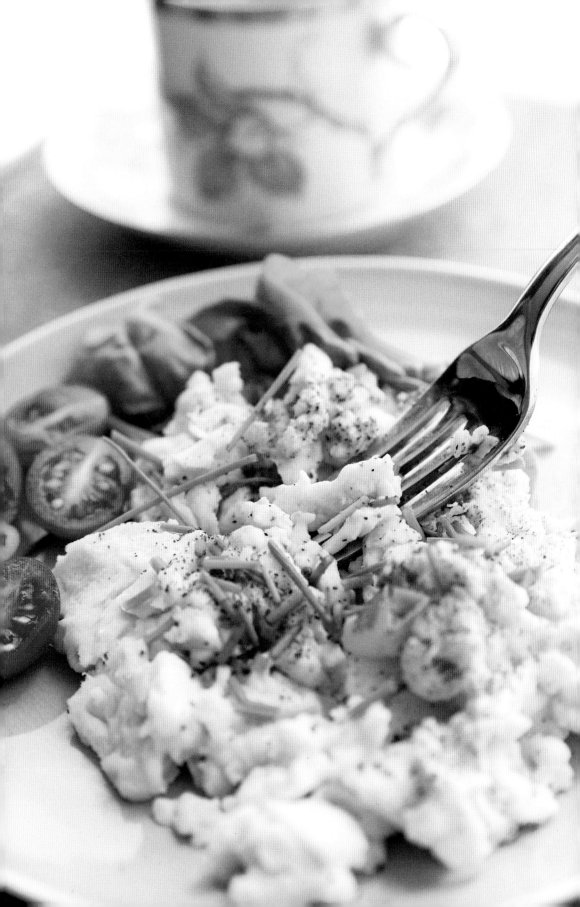

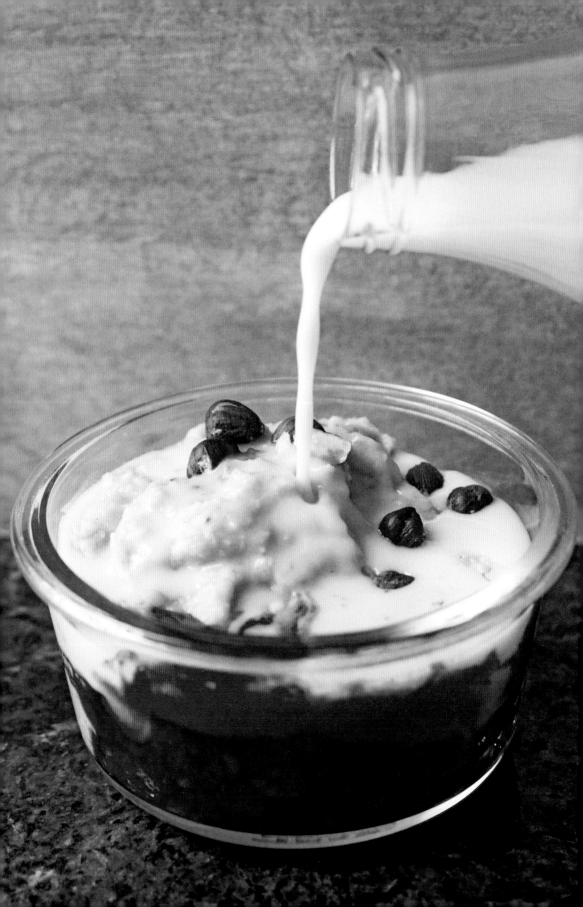

BANANA PORRIDGE WITH TANGY RASPBERRIES

My mom makes this for me when we have breakfast together. It is a variation on the classic porridge recipe with added bananas and raspberries. It does not take much longer to make than ordinary porridge and it feels unbelievably luxurious.

METHOD:
Take the raspberries out of the freezer and allow them to defrost for a few minutes at room temperature. Bring the oats, water, and some salt to a simmer on the stovetop. Mash the banana with a fork and stir it into the porridge towards the end of cooking.

Put the raspberries in the bottom of a bowl and pour the hot porridge over it. Serve with cold milk and hazelnuts.

You can make the porridge just as easily in your microwave, but I think it tastes that little bit better made on the stovetop.

Makes one portion

1¼ oz / 35 g rolled oats
1 cup / 250 ml water
salt
1 ripe banana
1 oz / 25 g frozen
  raspberries

To serve:
milk of your choice
hazelnuts

AVOCADO YOGHURT WITH PEACH

Makes one portion

1 large ripe avocado
½ frozen banana or
   similar volume of
   frozen berries
3½ tbsp / 50 ml rice milk
1 tbsp freshly-squeezed
   lemon juice
1 tsp honey
1 tsp vanilla powder

To serve:
peach
shelled hemp seeds

This green yogurt has a creamy, soft consistency and is quick to make. Perfect as breakfast or a snack if you want an alternative to dairy products.

METHOD:
Blend all the ingredients using a stick blender, and serve with fruit, seeds, or granola (see recipe on page 92).

Did you know?

Avocado has anti-inflammatory properties and contains large amounts of minerals, antioxidants, and vitamin E, which keeps the skin healthy and soft. It is also filling due to its high healthy omega-3 fat content.

Tip

If I have any ripe bananas in the house, I usually slice them up and freeze them in bags. They make the perfect base for smoothies and give this avocado yogurt a lovely sweetness.

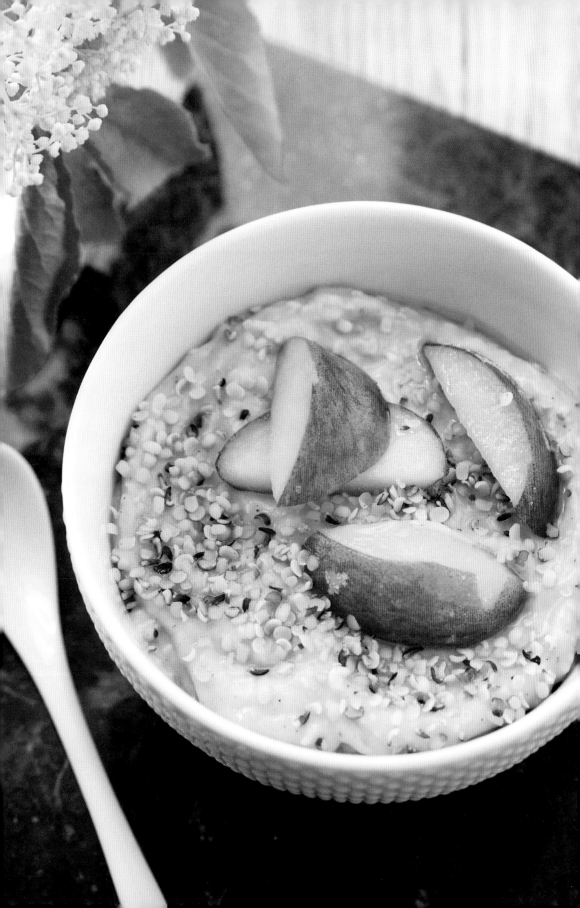

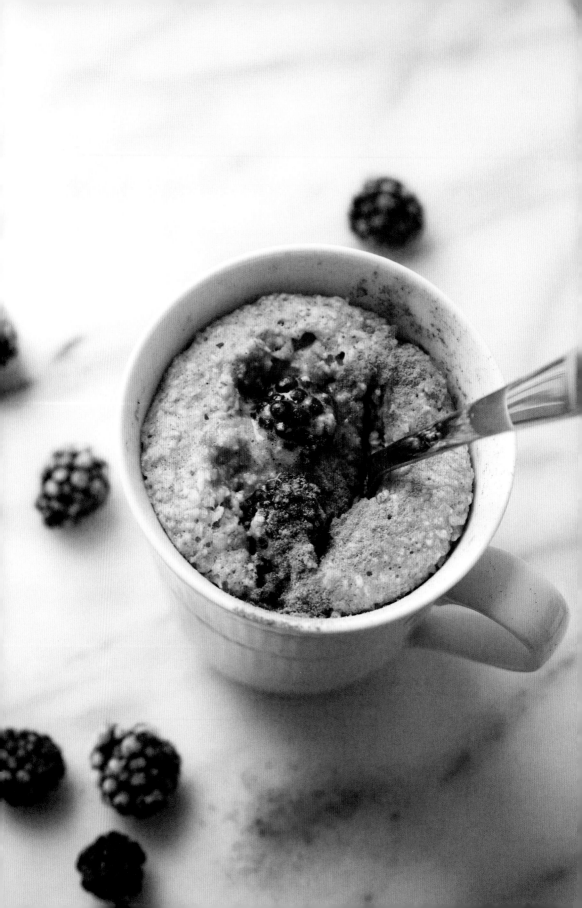

OAT, BANANA, AND BLACKBERRY MUG CAKE

Breakfast in a mug! A mug cake is the perfect breakfast when you don't have much time. It can be made quickly in your microwave and you can vary the recipe depending on the fruit and berries you have in the house.

METHOD:

Blend the oats, egg, and banana with a stick blender. Mix in the chopped nuts, blackberries, cinnamon, and shredded coconut. Grease a tall mug with coconut oil and pour in the mixture. Cook in your microwave for 1½ minutes on full power.

Makes one portion

1¼ oz / 35 g rolled oats
1 egg
½ banana
1 tbsp chopped hazelnuts
2 tbsp frozen blackberries
pinch ground cinnamon
1 tbsp shredded coconut
1 tsp cold-pressed coconut oil

COCONUT MILK, STRAWBERRY, AND CINNAMON SMOOTHIE

Makes one glass

generous ¾ cup /
  200 ml coconut milk
2 oz / 60 g frozen
  strawberries
1 tsp ground cinnamon
½ tsp vanilla powder

With a tin of coconut milk in your pantry, or another milk of your choice in the fridge, and berries in the freezer, you will always be able to quickly put together a delicious smoothie even if time is short.

METHOD:
Blend all the ingredients in a blender, adding more coconut milk if needed until you have the required consistency. Pour into a glass and enjoy ice-cold.

MANGO, BANANA, AND COCONUT SMOOTHIE

Makes one glass

generous ¾ cup /
  200 ml coconut milk
1 banana
2½ oz / 70 g frozen
  mango
1 tsp shredded coconut

METHOD:
Blend all the ingredients in a blender, adding more coconut milk as necessary to achieve the desired consistency. Pour into a glass and enjoy ice-cold.

OAT, BANANA, AND PEANUT BUTTER SMOOTHIE

Makes one glass

generous ¾ cup /
  200 ml oat milk
1 banana
¾ oz / 20 g rolled oats
1 tbsp peanut butter
½ tsp vanilla powder

METHOD:
Blend all the ingredients in a blender, adding more liquid as necessary to achieve the desired consistency. Pour into a glass and enjoy ice-cold.

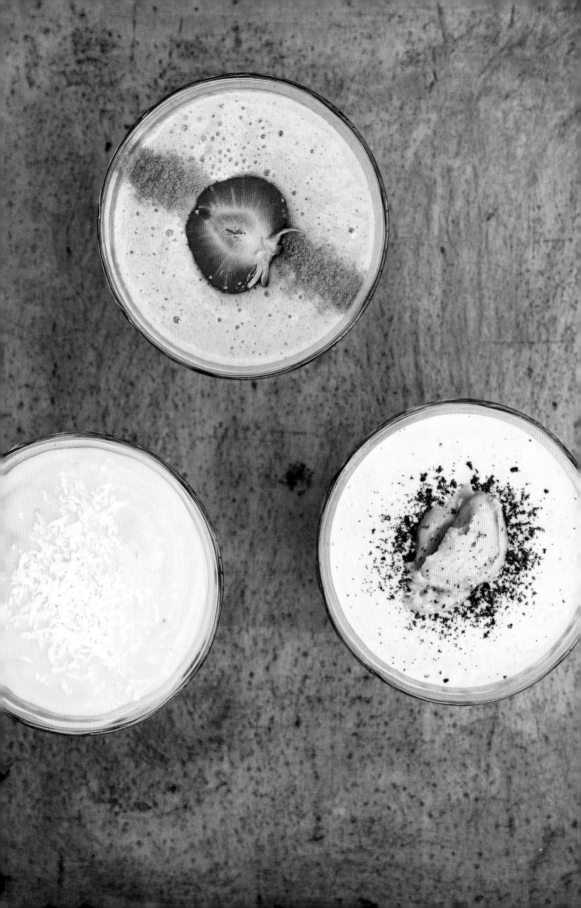

ULTRA-SPEEDY MICROWAVE NUT BREAD

Makes one loaf

1 egg

1¾ oz / 50 g nut flour,
   e.g. hazelnut flour or
   almond flour

½ tsp bread spice
   (e.g. aniseed, fennel,
   caraway)

½ tsp baking powder

salt

Freshly-baked bread for breakfast? This tasty breakfast bread can be made in just two minutes. Too good to be true? Try it for yourself!

METHOD:

Put all the ingredients in a bowl and mix with a fork. Transfer the mixture to a small, deep dish or to a plate. Cook in your microwave for two minutes on full power. Serve with nut butter, sliced fruit, berries, egg, or avocado.

Tip

It's easy to make your own nut flour by pulsing nuts in a food processor. Hazelnut flour produces a slightly nuttier bread, while almond flour will give your bread a slightly milder flavor.

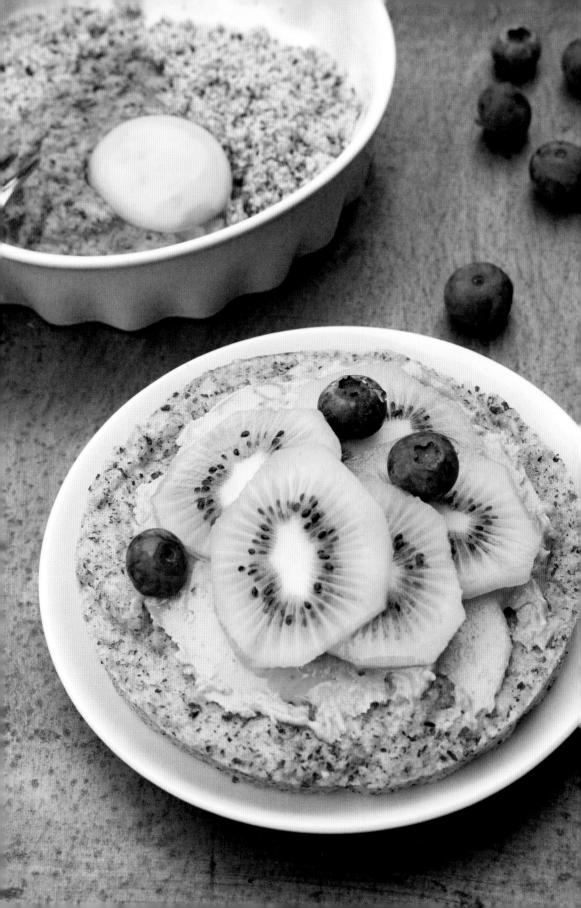

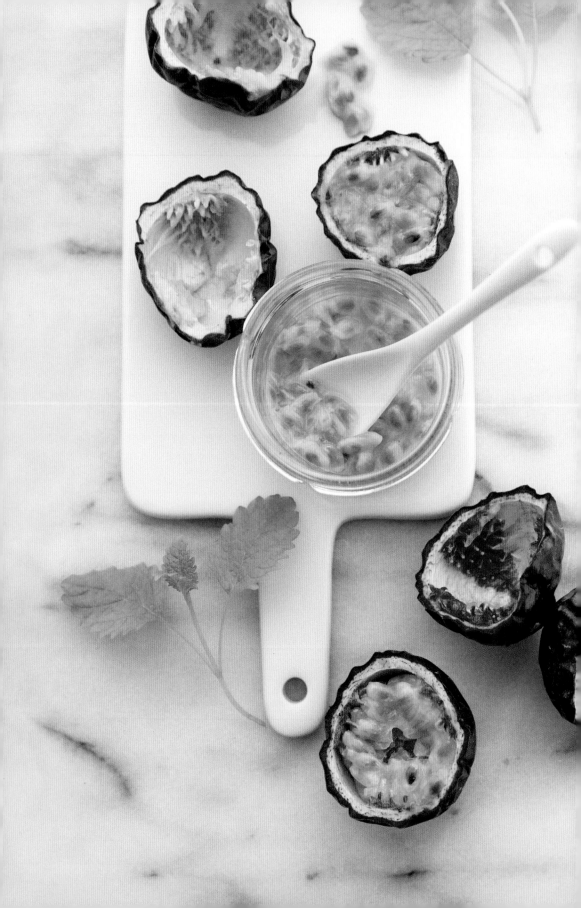

Breakfasts to prepare in advance

IF YOU'RE SOMEONE WHO LIKES to hit the snooze button in the morning, it can be hard work having to think about breakfast even before you have opened your eyes. But that is no reason to skip breakfast! When I have to get up early in the morning, I do most of the preparation the night before, making a quick breakfast that I can just take out of the fridge.

This chapter contains recipes for breakfasts that you can prepare fast. They are so easy that they almost make themselves while you are asleep. Set aside a bit of time in the evening, and you will thank yourself come the morning.

Do you eat your breakfast in a rush, with one foot in the kitchen and the other already outside the front door? It takes about 20 minutes for your body to feel full, so try to find the time to sit down and eat your breakfast in peace and quiet. A good breakfast lays the foundation for the rest of the day, and your body will be grateful for it.

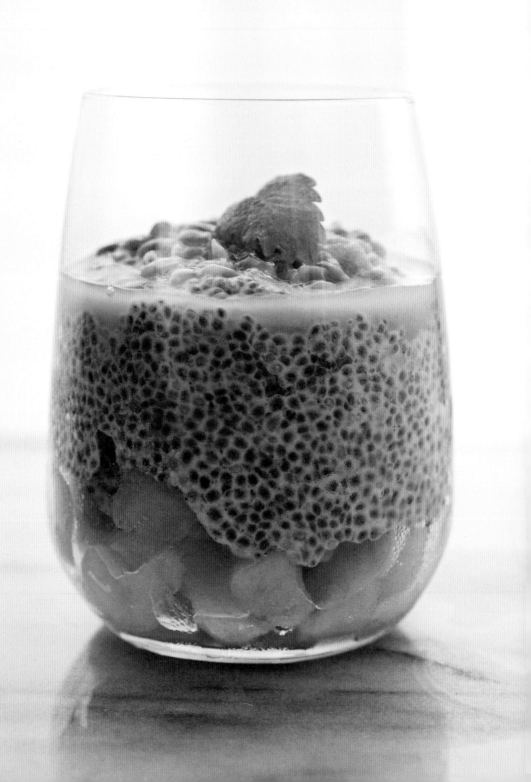

TROPICAL CHIA CREAM WITH MANGO AND PASSION FRUIT

Chia cream is the perfect breakfast to prepare the night before. The best thing about it is that it takes less than two minutes to put together in the evening and then makes itself in the fridge overnight.

METHOD:
Mix together the milk, chia seeds (the amount depends on the consistency you want), and vanilla powder in a bowl or glass jar with a lid. Do not leave any dry seeds on the surface. Place in the fridge for a few hours, ideally overnight. Remove from the fridge, give the mixture a stir, and mix in diced mango and passion fruit.

Did you know?

Chia seeds are real superseeds. They contain essential amino acids and as much protein as nuts, and are rich in minerals such as magnesium, calcium, phosphorus, and zinc. Perfect for blending into a smoothie, adding to porridge, or sprinkling onto yogurt.

Makes one portion

generous ¾ cup /
  200 ml coconut milk or
  milk of your choice
2–3 tbsp chia seeds
½ tsp vanilla powder
7 tbsp / 100 ml fresh or
  defrosted mango
1 passion fruit

CHOCOLATE CHIA CREAM

Makes one portion

Step 1:
generous ¾ cup /
  200 ml coconut milk
2–3 tbsp chia seeds

Step 2:
1 banana
2 tbsp raw cacao powder

Topping:
freeze-dried
  strawberries
banana
peanut butter
coconut cream
cacao nibs
chia seeds

Chocolate cream for breakfast? Oh yes you can! This is a fun way to ring the changes with your chia cream. Blending the chia cream with banana at the end gives it a less viscous consistency, and the banana and cacao flavors work perfectly together.

METHOD:
Step 1: Mix the coconut milk and chia seeds (the amount depends on the consistency you want) so that the seeds swell in the milk. Place in the fridge for a few hours, ideally overnight.

Step 2: Blend the chia cream in the blender with the banana and raw cacao powder. Top with some of the following: freeze-dried strawberries, banana, peanut butter, coconut cream, or cacao nibs.

Did you know?

Cacao nibs are pure chocolate made from cocoa beans that have been crushed into small pieces. They have a mild cocoa taste and can be used in a variety of ways including in smoothies, coffee, and desserts.

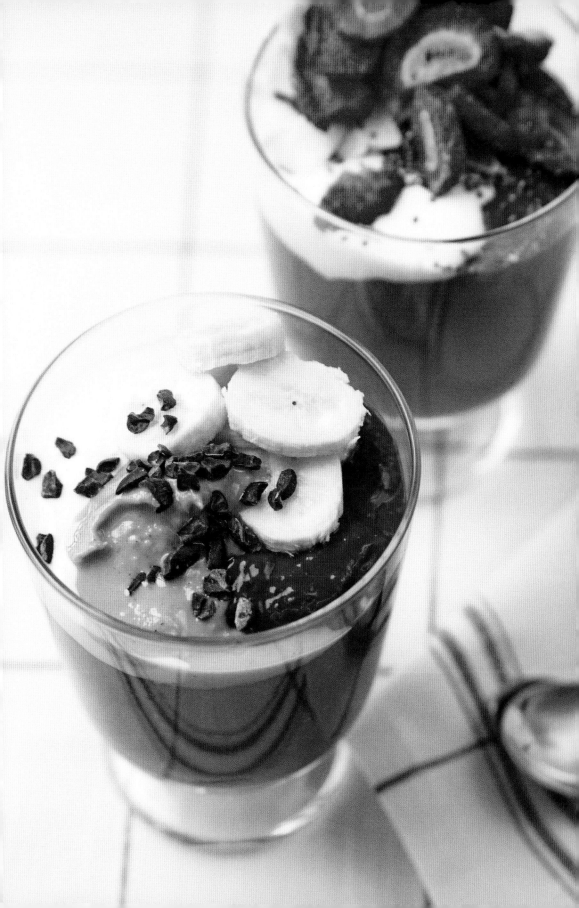

RAW QUINOA PORRIDGE WITH BLUEBERRIES

Makes one portion

½ cup / 100 g quinoa

1¼ cups / 300 ml water

1 banana

1 tsp ground cinnamon

½ tsp ground cardamom

½ tsp vanilla powder

To serve:

1 oz / 30 g defrosted blueberries

½ peach

A chilled porridge that is easily prepared the night before. Quinoa is a plant that is naturally gluten-free. It contains slow carbohydrates that keep hunger at bay for a long time and provide lots of energy. It is also a complete source of protein, so if you eat a lot of vegetarian food quinoa will help you get the protein you need. You only need a blender and a minute to prepare it the night before, and you are there.

METHOD:

Soak the quinoa in the water and place it in the fridge overnight. In the morning, drain off the water and rinse the quinoa with fresh water. Blend the quinoa with the banana into a smooth porridge and add the spices. You may want to add a splash of water depending on your preferred consistency. Serve with defrosted blueberries and sliced peach.

Did you know?

Blueberries are full of antioxidants that protect our cells from premature ageing. They are also good for your sight and contain minerals such as potassium, phosphorus, calcium, and magnesium.

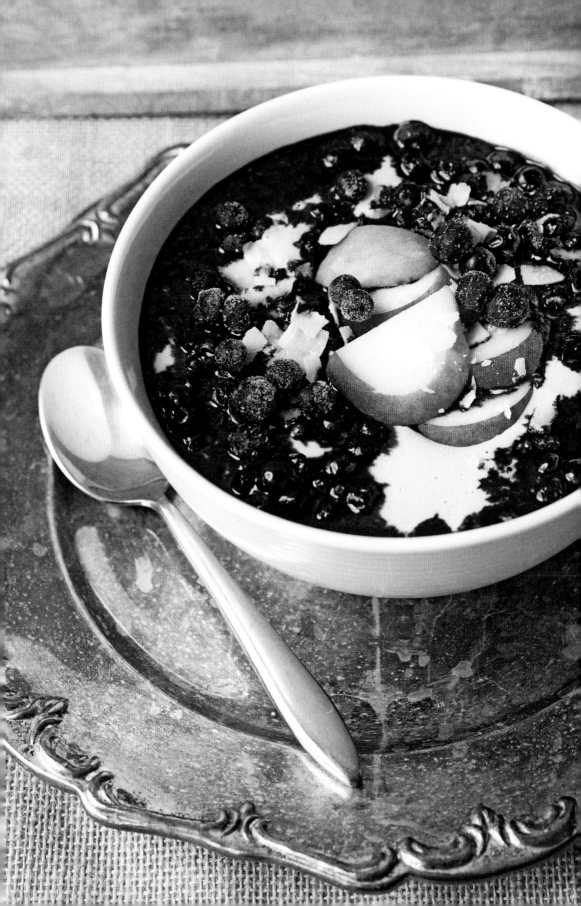

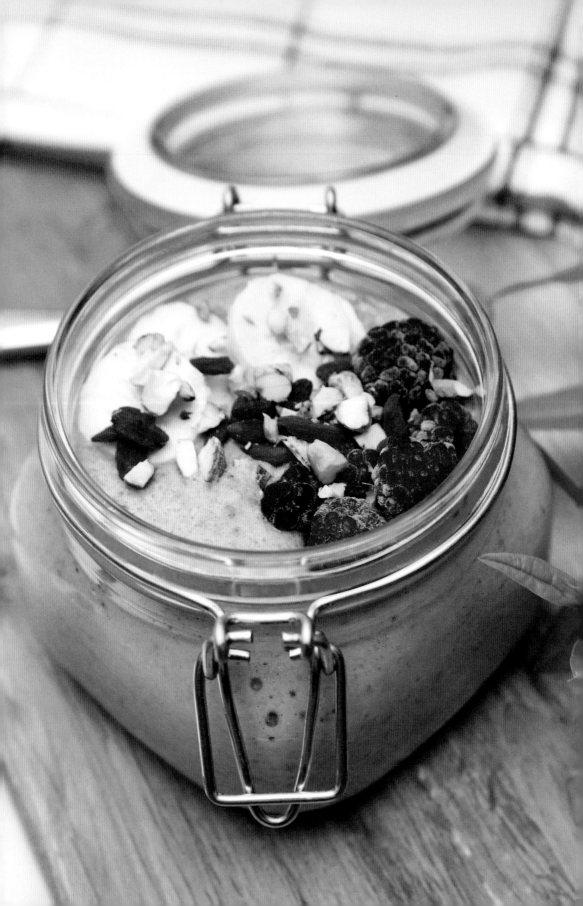

CHILLED BUCKWHEAT PORRIDGE WITH BANANA AND RASPBERRIES

This is one of my absolute favorite breakfasts. It takes no time to prepare the porridge in the evening, and you can easily take it to work in a glass jar with a lid. I have used banana and raspberries in this version, but you can just as easily use your own favorite berries according to season and taste.

METHOD:
Soak the buckwheat and sunflower seeds in 1¼ cups / 300 ml water overnight. Rinse the buckwheat and sunflower seeds thoroughly and blend together with the other ingredients. You can also mix in a scoop of protein powder of your choice. It will add taste and texture and keep hunger at bay a little longer.

Serve with berries, fruit, and some seeds and/or nuts.

Makes one portion

2½ oz / 75 g whole buckwheat
1¾ oz / 50 g sunflower seeds
1¼ cups / 300 ml water
1¾ oz / 50 g raspberries
½ banana
3½ tbsp / 50 ml rice milk
½ tsp ground cinnamon
protein powder if liked

Topping:
berries and fruit
seeds and nuts

GRANOLA WITH NUTS AND DRIED FRUIT

Makes one trayful

Dry ingredients:

2½ oz / 70 g rolled oats

3½ oz / 100 g sunflower
  seeds

2 oz / 55 g chopped nuts,
  e.g. cashews, almonds

2½ oz / 75 g dried fruit,
  e.g. dates, figs, raisins

1¼ oz / 35 g pumpkin
  seeds

2 tbsp whole flaxseeds

2 tbsp ground cinnamon

1 tsp sea salt flakes

Wet ingredients:

2 tbsp cold-pressed
  coconut oil

2 tbsp peanut butter

2 tbsp honey

2 tbsp water

Breakfast becomes that bit more tasty and luxurious with home-made granola. This is a good base recipe that can be adapted to your preferences or to what you have in your pantry, and it is really quick to prepare in the evening. This recipe makes enough granola for the whole week. It is nice sprinkled over a smoothie in the morning and makes a welcome gift for someone you love.

METHOD:

Heat the oven to 360 °F / 180 °C. Put all the dry ingredients into a bowl and mix. Melt the coconut oil in the microwave and mix it with the peanut butter, honey, and a splash of water. Stir this mixture into the dry ingredients and mix well.

Spread it out onto a baking tray covered with parchment paper and bake in the middle of the oven for 12–15 minutes. Remove and check whether the granola is crunchy; if not, return it to the oven for another minute or so. Take care not to let it burn. Allow to cool and store in a jar with a lid.

Tip

For a nut-free granola, replace the nuts with seeds and the peanut butter with tahini.

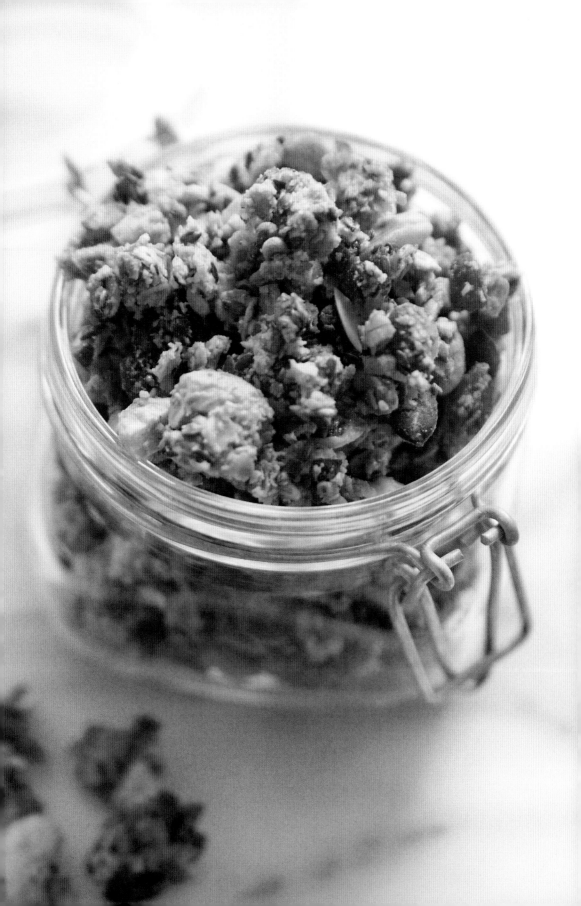

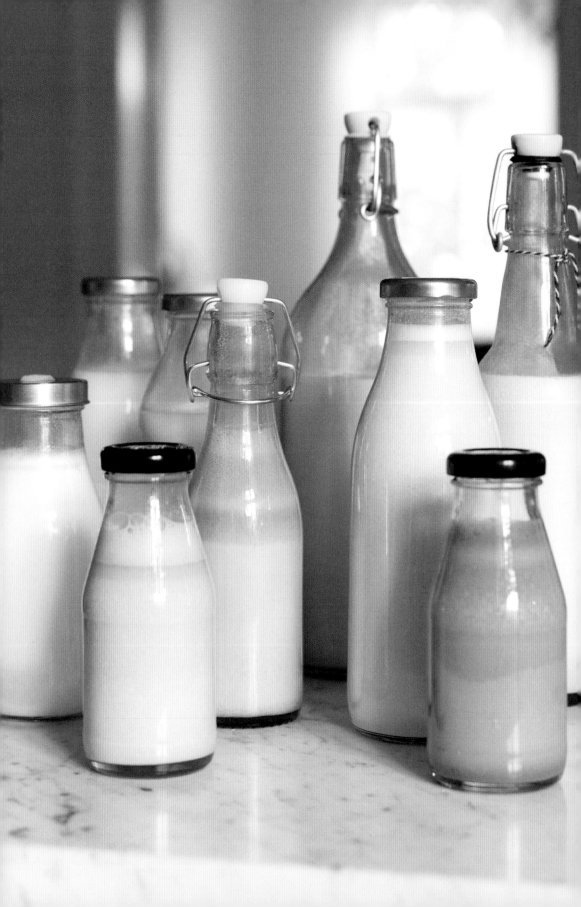

NUT AND SEED DRINKS

Homemade nut drinks are as delicious as they come and store-bought varieties cannot compare either in taste or in nutritional content. They are also really easy and so much more fun to make yourself. Experiment with different seeds, nuts, and flavorings—here are a few of my favorites.

METHOD:
Blend the nuts, seeds, coconut, or oats with the cold water for three minutes. Add any sweeteners or flavorings and blend for another minute. Strain the milk through a nut milk bag and store in a bottle sealed with a cork.

The drink will keep in the fridge for two or three days.

Tip

If you are using nuts, soak them and put them in a cool place, ideally the fridge, for at least six hours. This eliminates hard-to-digest enzymes and gives the milk a milder taste. Then rinse the nuts well before blending them with some fresh water. The nut pulp left over is excellent for raw food balls or bread-making.

Base recipe— makes one quart / liter

1 quart / 1 liter water, or less, depending on how thick you want your milk to be

1¼ cups / 300 ml of either nuts, hemp seeds, shredded coconut, or rolled oats

2 tbsp neutral cold-pressed oil, e.g. coconut oil, rapeseed oil

small pinch sea salt flakes

Sweeteners:
4–5 fresh dates, pitted, or 1 tbsp honey

Flavorings:
cinnamon, cardamom, matcha, raw cacao powder, or turmeric

HERE ARE SOME OF MY FAVORITES:

HAZELNUT MILK WITH CINNAMON AND DATES

1 quart / 1 liter water
7 oz / 195 g hazelnuts
5 fresh dates, pitted
2 tsp cold-pressed coconut oil
1 tsp ground cinnamon
½ tsp ground cardamom
small pinch sea salt flakes

CHOCOLATE MILK

1 quart / 1 liter water
7 oz / 195 g hazelnuts
5 fresh dates, pitted
2 tsp cold-pressed coconut oil
1 tbsp raw cacao powder
small pinch sea salt flakes

ALMOND MILK

1 quart / 1 liter water
7½ oz / 210 g almonds
2 tsp cold-pressed rapeseed oil
1 tsp vanilla powder
small pinch sea salt flakes

ALMOND MILK WITH MATCHA

1 quart / 1 liter water
7½ oz / 210 g almonds
2 tsp honey
2 tsp cold-pressed rapeseed oil
½ tbsp matcha powder

ALMOND MILK WITH TURMERIC

1 quart / 1 liter water
7½ oz / 210 g almonds
2 tsp honey
2 tsp cold-pressed rapeseed oil
2 tsp dried ground turmeric

OAT MILK

1 quart / 1 liter water
3½ oz / 105 g rolled oats
2 tsp honey
2 tsp cold-pressed rapeseed oil
small pinch sea salt flakes

HEMP SEED MILK WITH CACAO

1 quart / 1 liter water
4½ oz / 125 g shelled hemp seeds
5 fresh dates, pitted
½ tbsp raw cacao powder
2 tsp cold-pressed rapeseed oil
1 tsp vanilla powder
1 tsp ground cinnamon
small pinch sea salt flakes

COCONUT MILK

1 quart / 1 liter water
3½ oz / 105 g shredded coconut
2 tsp cold-pressed coconut oil
small pinch sea salt flakes

CASHEW MILK

1 quart / 1 liter water
6½ oz / 180 g cashew nuts
2 tsp cold-pressed rapeseed oil
small pinch sea salt flakes

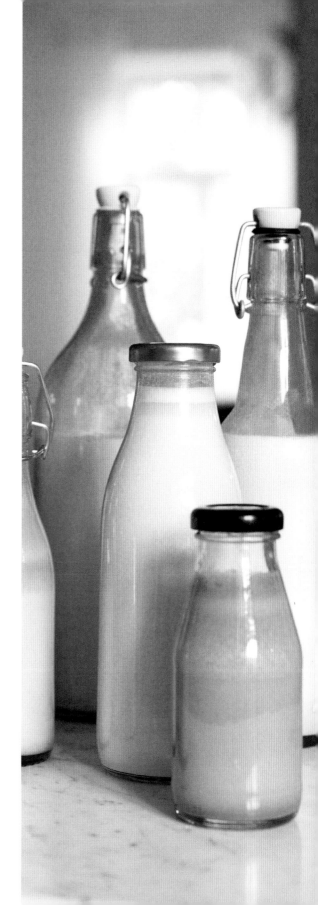

SEEDED CRISPBREAD

Makes one trayful

3½ oz / 100 g sunflower
   seeds

2½ oz / 70 g pumpkin
   seeds

2 oz / 60 g sesame seeds

1 oz / 25 g shelled hemp
   seeds

1 oz / 30 g whole
   flaxseeds

2 tbsp chia seeds

1 tbsp cold-pressed
   rapeseed oil

1 cup / 250 ml hot
   water

½ tsp salt or
   herb salt

Seeded crispbread is perhaps the simplest bread you can possibly bake. It is healthy, cheap, tasty, and almost ridiculously easy to make. I often make a trayful during the week and eat it for breakfast, as a snack, or to go with soup or a salad.

METHOD:
Heat the oven to 360 °F / 180 °C. Mix all the dry ingredients apart from the salt and then add the oil and hot water. Stir and allow to stand for a minute or two. Cover a baking tray with parchment paper and spread out the mixture in a thin layer. Sprinkle with a little herb salt or ordinary salt. Bake in the center of the oven for about 25 minutes.

Seeded crispbread is best kept in a dry place or in the fridge, where it will keep for about a week.

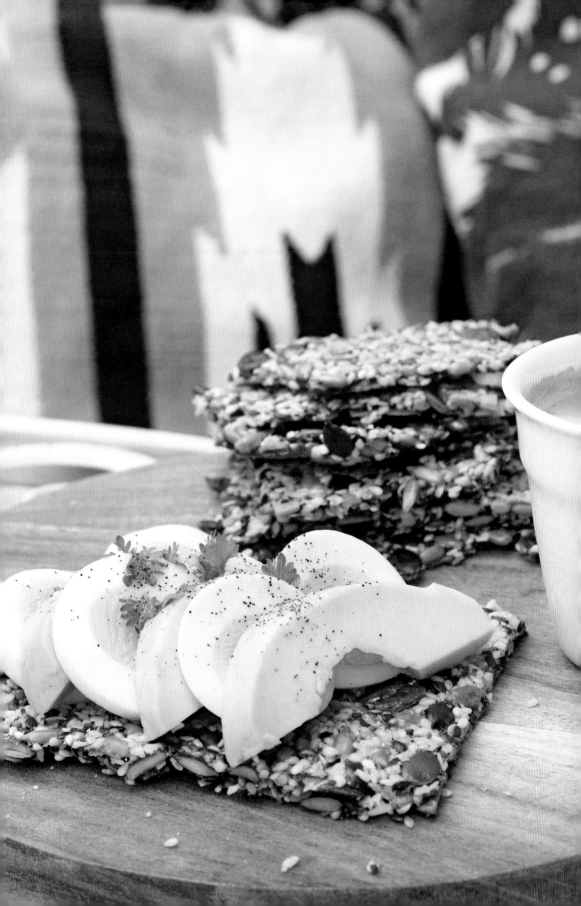

OVERNIGHT OATS WITH APPLE

Makes one portion

⅔ cup / 150 ml rice milk
1¼ oz / 35 g rolled oats
½ apple, grated
1 tbsp flaxseeds
½ tsp ground cinnamon
salt

Topping:
fresh fruit or berries,
  nuts, seeds, crispy
  coconut biscuits,
  or chia jam

Overnight oats are the ultimate working breakfast. It can be quickly prepared the night before and varied in a multitude of ways. The base consists of a grain such as rolled oats or buckwheat flakes, and milk. Flavor to taste and place in the fridge to swell overnight. In the morning you'll have a ready-made porridge that you can top with nuts, seeds, fruit, berries, or perhaps even chia jam (see recipe on page 132).

METHOD:
Put all the ingredients into a bowl and mix. Transfer into a glass jar with a lid and store in the fridge overnight. In the morning, remove your porridge and top with fresh fruit, berries, or seeds etc.

OVERNIGHT OATS WITH CARROT

Makes one portion

⅔ cup / 150 ml almond
  milk
2½ oz / 75 g buckwheat
  flakes
½ carrot, grated
1 tbsp chia seeds
½ tsp ground cinnamon
½ tsp ground
  cardamom
salt

Topping:
fresh fruit or berries,
nuts, seeds, crispy
coconut biscuits,
or chia jam

METHOD:
Put all the ingredients into a bowl and mix. Transfer into a glass jar with a lid and store in the fridge overnight. In the morning, remove your porridge and top with fresh fruit, berries, or seeds etc.

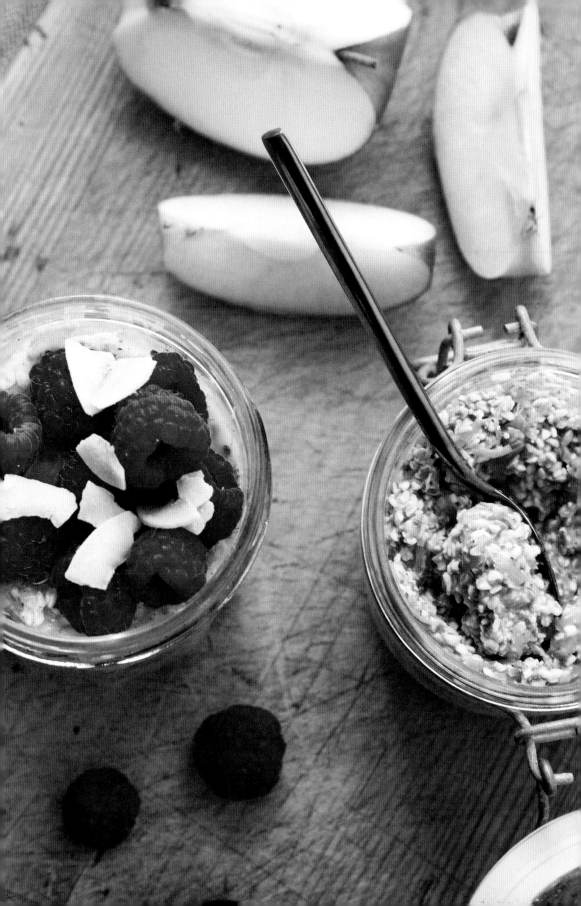

BLUEBERRY CREAM WITH CHIA SEEDS

Makes one portion

2 oz / 60 g blueberries,
  fresh or frozen
7 tbsp / 100 ml water
2 tbsp chia seeds
1–2 tsp honey
pinch vanilla powder

To serve:
fresh blueberries
coconut cream
mint

A delicious and healthy blueberry cream that is full of energy. Soaking the chia seeds creates a gelatinous film of dietary fibers that help maintain bowel health.

METHOD:
Defrost any frozen blueberries you are using. Using a jar blender or stick blender, blend all the ingredients into a smooth cream. Place in the fridge for at least an hour, or overnight, and serve with fresh blueberries, coconut cream, and mint.

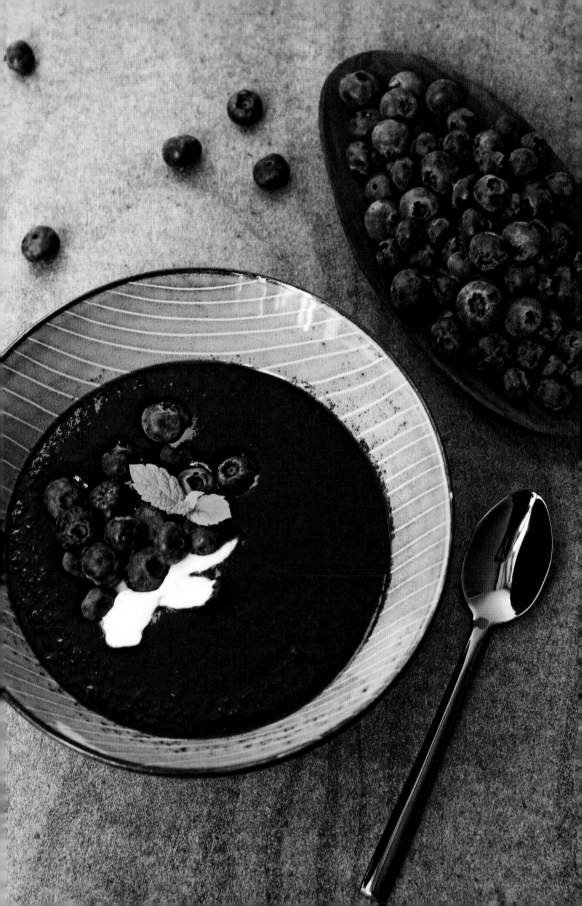

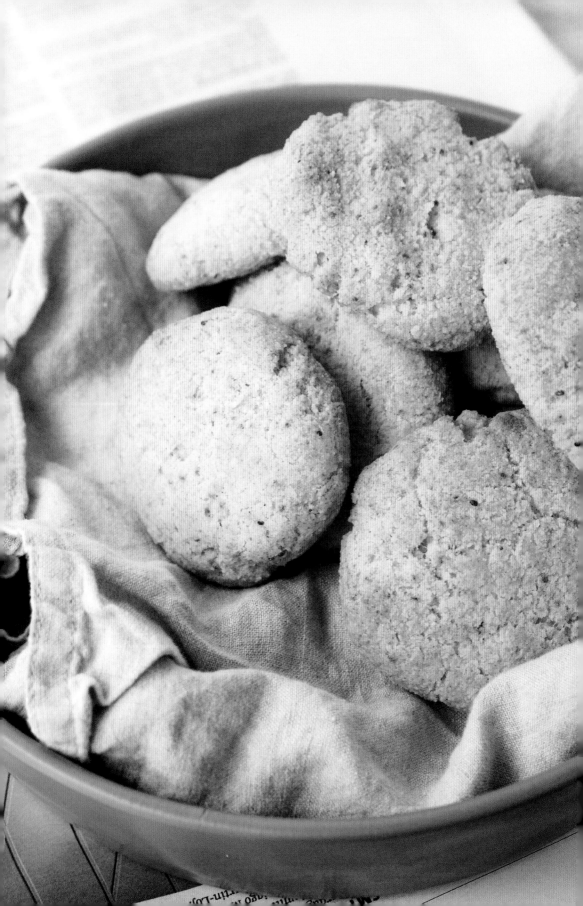

ALMOND SCONES

Making scones is a really quick and simple way to enjoy the pleasures of baked goods fresh from the oven. My scones are made from almond flour, which makes them moist and filling. Prepare everything the night before by putting all the dry ingredients into a bowl and mixing. In the morning, just add almond milk, coconut oil, and egg, and bake the scones in the oven while you are getting ready.

METHOD:

Heat the oven to 390 °F / 200 °C. Mix the flour, psyllium husk, baking powder, and salt in a food processor (you can prepare in advance up to this point). Add the almond milk, coconut oil, egg, and chia seeds and stir to make a smooth dough. Let it rest for five minutes so that it swells a little. The dough will be sticky, but it will come right in the oven. Drop small balls of the dough onto a baking tray covered with parchment paper. Bake in the middle of the oven for 10–15 minutes.

Makes eight small scones or two large ones

1⅔ cups / 400 ml almond flour
1 tbsp psyllium husk
2 tsp baking powder
½ tsp salt
⅔ cup / 150 ml unsweetened almond milk
7 tbsp / 100 ml cold-pressed coconut oil
1 egg
1 tbsp chia seeds

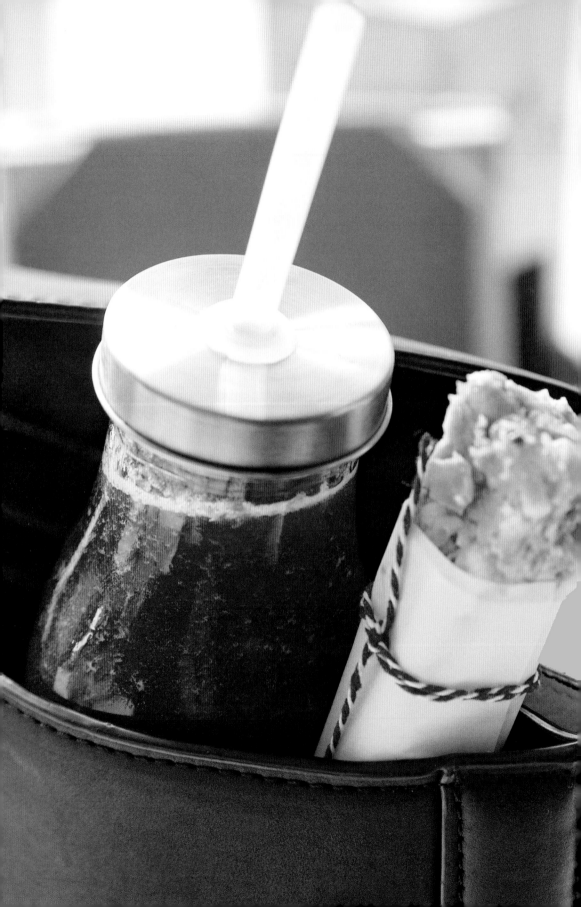

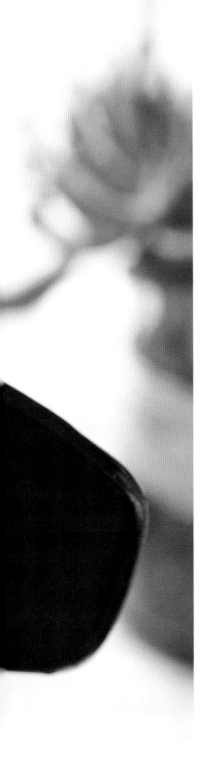

Breakfast on the go

SOME DAYS THERE JUST IS NOT TIME to sit down and eat breakfast in peace and quiet. Perhaps you commute, and spend your morning on a bus or train or in a car? Or do you need something you can easily eat while walking to work? Maybe there's not enough time or you don't feel hungry first thing in the morning?

To make sure your energy levels do not slump and you retain your sunny mood as the morning wears on, it is a good idea to take breakfast with you to eat on the way or when you get to work.

One tip is to invest in good bottles and packaging that make it easy for you to take your breakfast with you without having to take half the kitchen along with you.

Here are some suggestions that will hopefully give you some inspiration.

CRANBERRY BREAKFAST BITES

Makes six or seven bites

1¼ oz / 35 g rolled oats

¾ oz / 20 g shredded
   coconut

1 oz / 25 g almonds,
   chopped

2 tbsp dried cranberries,
   chopped

½ tsp vanilla powder

½ tsp ground cinnamon

salt

1 ripe banana

2 tsp honey

Sweet little breakfast biscuits that are perfect when you are on the go. Make a double batch and freeze them, so that you have some ready to hand when time is short.

METHOD:
Heat the oven to 360 °F / 180 °C. Put everything except the banana and the honey into a bowl, mix, then add the mashed banana and honey. Make the mixture into small balls using your hands and place them on a baking tray covered with parchment paper. Bake in the middle of the oven for 15–20 minutes until they are golden brown.

Tip

Dried cranberries sold in ordinary food stores often contain large amounts of white sugar. Look for cranberries that are sweetened with apple or pineapple juice, a slightly healthier option that is just as delicious.

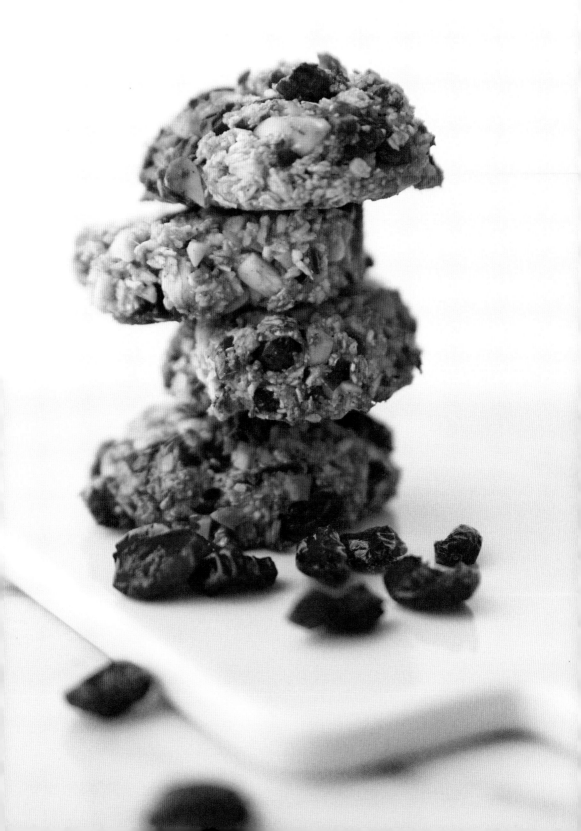

RAW PEANUT GRANOLA BARS

Makes four bars

1 scant cup / 100 g
  coarsely-chopped
  nuts, e.g. almonds and
  cashews
1¼ oz / 35 g rolled oats
1 tbsp sugarless peanut
  butter
1 tbsp cold-pressed
  coconut oil, melted
5 dried apricots
2 tsp honey
pinch salt

Satisfying bars with peanut butter and apricots that are high in energy. Making your own bars is really easy, and the best thing is that you can choose exactly what you want to have in them. This is a good base recipe to start with, and it easily be adapted to suit the contents of your pantry.

METHOD:

Chop the apricots coarsely. Put the nuts with the other ingredients into a bowl and stir until you have a sticky mixture. Using your hands, form the mixture into a square about ¾ in. / 2 cm high on a plate covered with parchment paper and put this into the fridge for at least an hour. Cut the square into four equal pieces.

These keep very well in the freezer.

Tip

I always buy organic peanut butter made only from roasted peanuts and a little sea salt. You'll find this in the jam and nut butter section in most food stores. Some brands contain large amounts of sugar, which I think is unnecessary, so I would advise you always to read the list of ingredients.

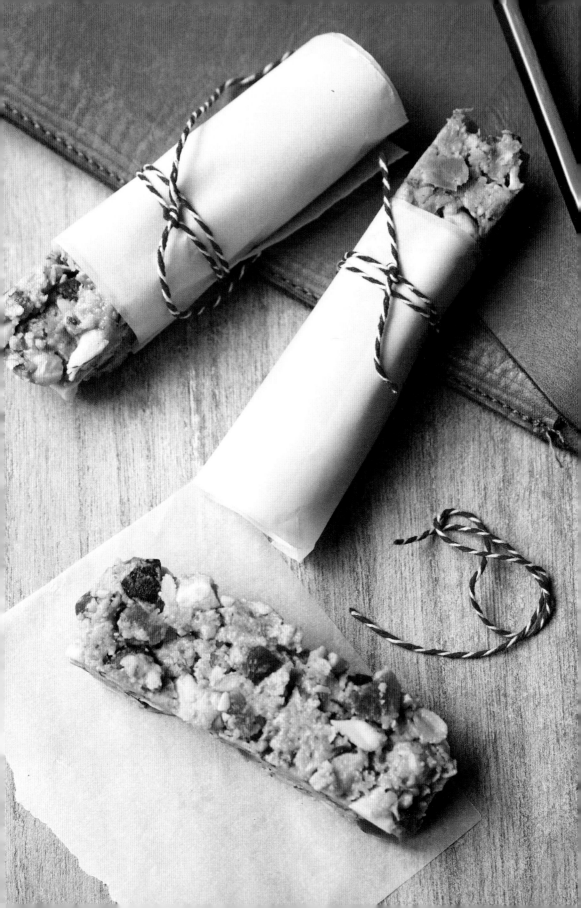

MATCHA CHIA GLOW

Makes one glass

generous ¾ cup /
  200 ml almond milk
7 tbsp / 100 ml water
2 tbsp chia seeds
1 tsp matcha powder
1 tsp honey
½ tsp vanilla powder
ice

I drank matcha chia glow for the first time when I was in New York, and became completely hooked. I decided I had to try and make my own version when I got home, and it quickly became one of my favorite recipes. The combination of matcha and chia provides a really satisfying, energizing breakfast in liquid form—perfect when you are on the go!

METHOD:

Put all the ingredients into a shaker or a glass and mix. Allow the drink to stand for about 15 minutes so that the chia seeds swell, and serve with ice.

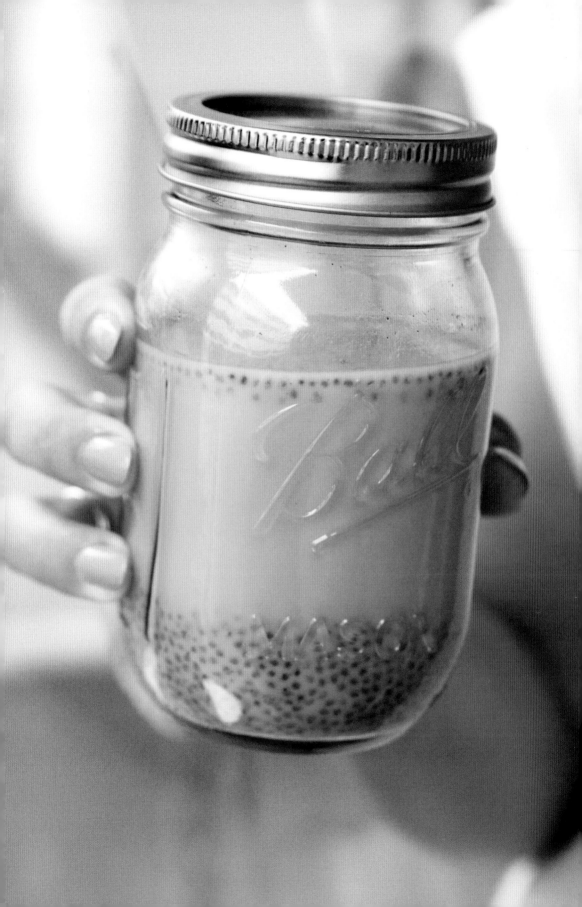

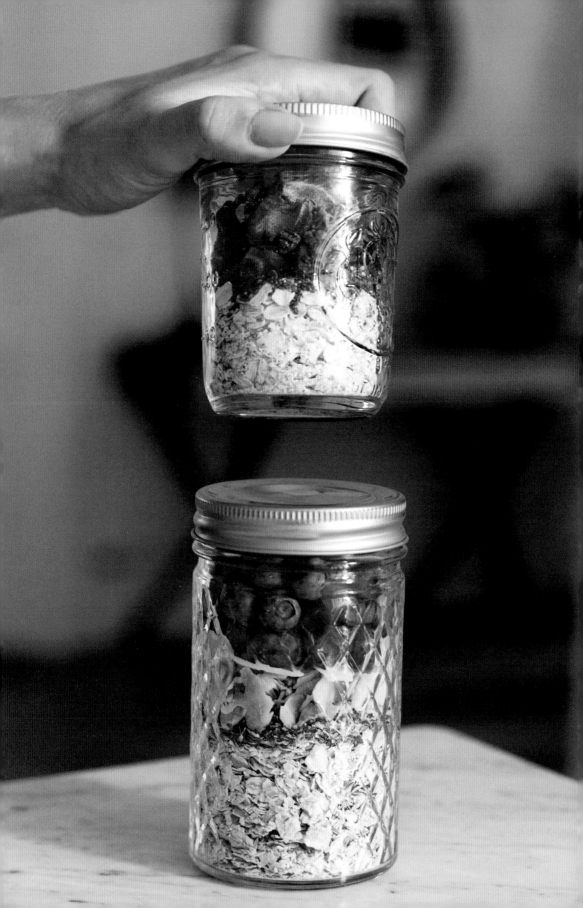

OATS IN A JAR

Here's a porridge that you can eat when and where you want. All you have to do is add water or milk and the porridge is ready. Perfect in your sports bag or when you're out on a trip! Use the base recipe below and mix in seeds, spices, dried berries, and nuts depending on what you fancy. The great thing is that you can prepare jars for the whole week and just throw one into your bag in the morning.

METHOD:
Mix all the ingredients together. When you are ready to eat the porridge, add ⅔ cup, or 150 ml, of cold or hot water, or milk of your choice. Mix well and allow to stand for eight to ten minutes. Add your favorite flavoring.

Makes
one portion

1¼ oz / 35 g rolled oats
1 tsp flaxseeds
1 tsp chia seeds
pinch ground cinnamon
pinch ground
  cardamom
salt

Flavorings:
crispy coconut biscuits,
  cacao nibs, freeze-
  dried berries, fresh
  berries, or nuts

BUCKWHEAT WRAPS WITH FRIED EGG

Makes four wraps

6½ oz / 190 g
  buckwheat flour
1 tbsp psyllium husk
½ tbsp chia seeds
salt
7 tbsp / 100 ml water
1½ tbsp cold-pressed
  coconut oil

Filling for each wrap:
1 tbsp tahini
1 fried egg
2 cocktail tomatoes
handful of baby spinach
¼ bell pepper
½ avocado
a little parsley
1 tsp olive oil

Satisfying buckwheat wraps filled with egg and vegetables. They are easy to fry in your frying pan, and perfect to take with you to the beach or on an outing.

METHOD:
Mix the dry ingredients into a fine flour, and then add the water and coconut oil. Mix into a smooth dough and divide into four equal pieces. Roll the dough out thinly on a floured surface and fry in a hot frying pan until the wraps have some color.

Filling: Spread the wraps with the tahini and then add the fried egg, vegetables, olive oil, and some salt and pepper. Fold up the wraps and roll into wax paper or parchment paper secured with string.

Did you know?

Please note that the amount of filling above is for a single wrap. The wraps will keep for two or three days in the fridge and can easily be heated up in the microwave.

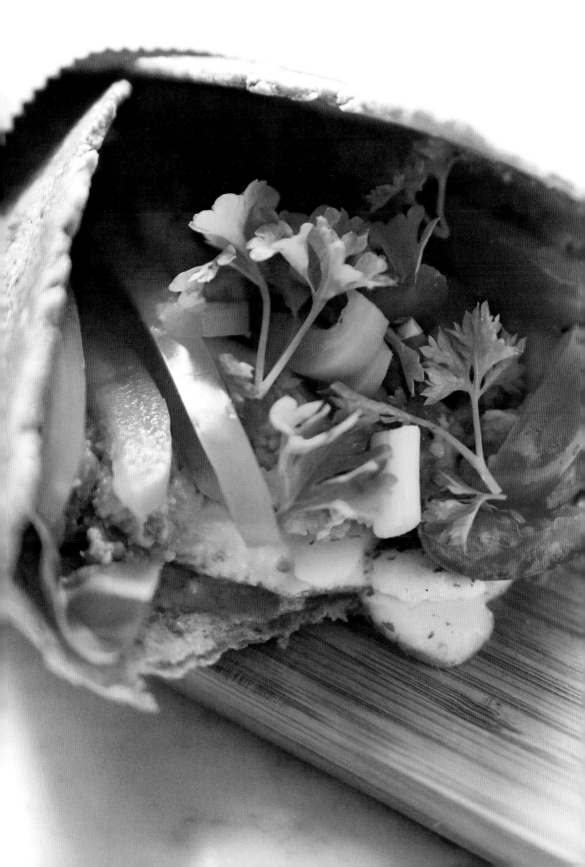

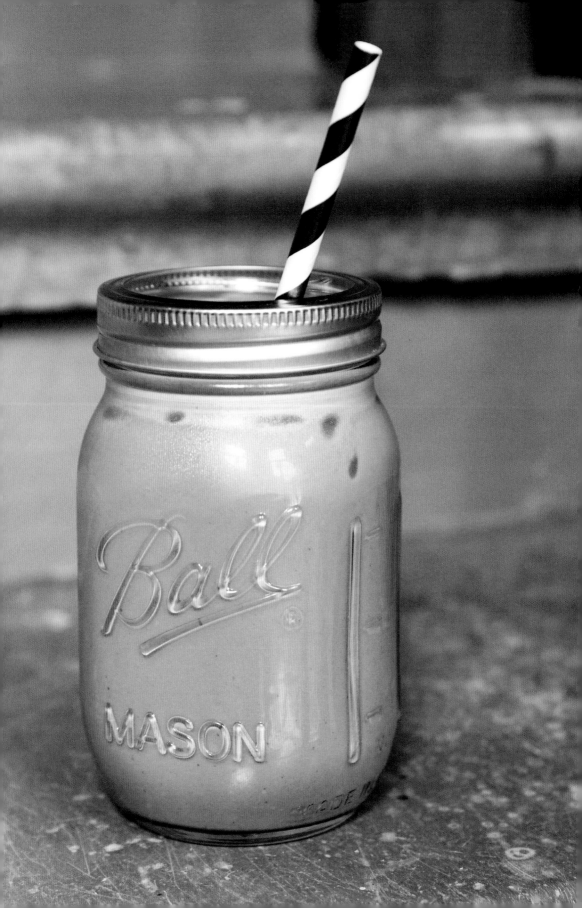

MOCHA BANANA BREAKFAST SMOOTHIE

Coffee and breakfast all in one—the perfect smoothie when you're on the go, it will wake you up and fill you up! The banana increases the feeling of fullness and gives the smoothie some natural sweetness.

METHOD:
Blend all the ingredients in a blender, adding more almond milk if needed. Pour into a glass bottle with a lid or another handy container that you can take with you to drink from on your way.

Enjoy ice-cold.

Makes one portion

1¼ cups / 300 ml almond milk
¾ oz / 20 g rolled oats
1 ripe banana
1 tbsp almond butter
1 tbsp raw cacao powder
2 fresh dates, pitted
1–2 tsp instant coffee to taste
ice

VANILLA AND COCONUT SMOOTHIE

Makes one portion

7 tbsp / 100 ml coconut water

7 tbsp / 100 ml coconut milk

½ frozen banana

2 fresh dates

¾ oz / 20 g shredded coconut

1 scoop protein powder, vanilla-flavored

pinch vanilla powder

pinch sea salt

ice

A creamy, protein-rich smoothie that satisfies, thanks to good fats contained in the coconut milk, the carbohydrates in the banana, and the protein powder. You can easily replace the protein powder with a vegetable alternative such as hemp or pea protein.

METHOD:
Blend all the ingredients in a blender, adding more liquid if needed. Pour into a bottle with a straw or a shaker and drink ice-cold.

BERRY AND BEET SMOOTHIE

Makes one portion

generous ¾ cup / 200 ml almond milk

1¾ oz / 50 g raspberries

1¾ oz / 50 g strawberries

1 beet, cooked

¾–1¼ in. / 2–3 cm fresh ginger

1 tsp honey

ice

A smoothie is the perfect breakfast when you are on the move. If you often eat breakfast on the go, one suggestion is to get some handy bottles to carry your smoothie in. There are suitable glass bottles with a hole for a straw (as in the picture on page 141), and shakers or ordinary water bottles also work well.

The Berry and Beet Smoothie is shown on page 106.

METHOD:
Blend all the ingredients in a blender, adding more liquid if needed. Pour into a bottle with a straw or a shaker and drink ice-cold.

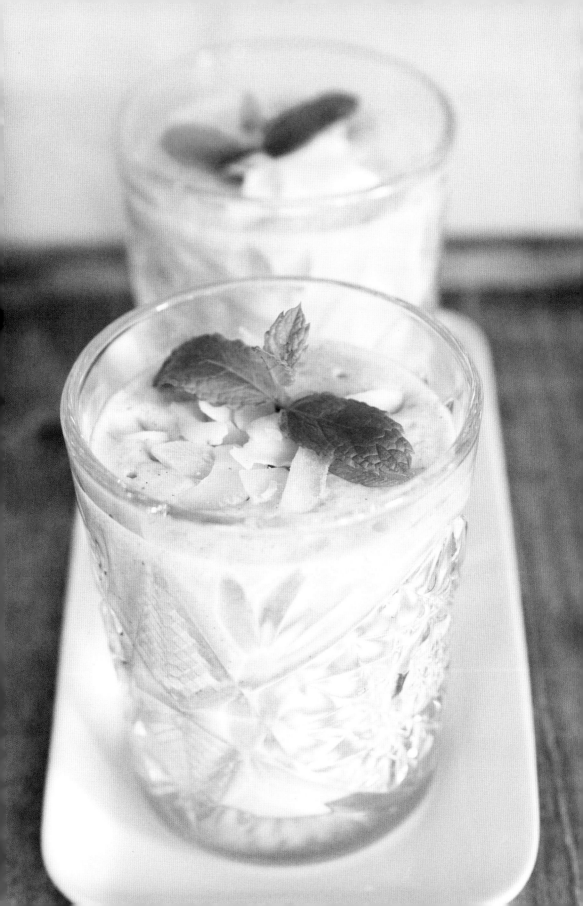

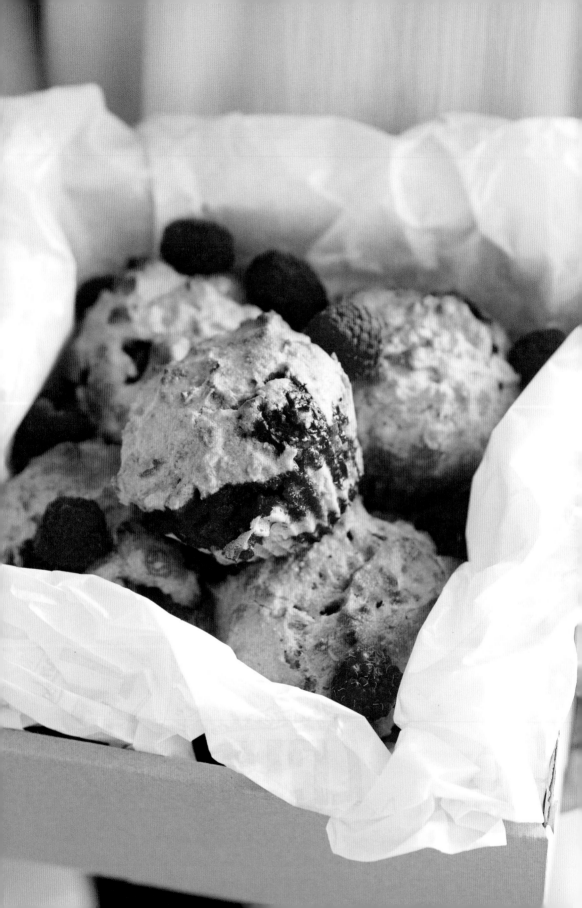

RASPBERRY AND CARDAMOM BREAKFAST MUFFINS

Delicious breakfast muffins flavored with raspberry and cardamom. Just as good whether you have them as a snack or enjoy them with your coffee at work.

METHOD:
Heat the oven to 350 °F / 175 °C. Blend the egg, banana, and melted coconut oil with a stick blender. Mix all the dry ingredients in a bowl and stir into the egg mixture. Continue to blend until smooth, stir in the raspberries (defrost frozen raspberries first), and then pour the mixture into muffin cases. Bake in the center of the oven for about 15 minutes.

Tip

Oat flour is available in most food stores, but you can just as easily make your own by pulsing rolled oats in a food processor until you have a fine flour. Oats are naturally gluten-free, but if you have celiac disease you should use guaranteed gluten-free oats, as there are sometimes traces of gluten in "ordinary" oats.

Solid coconut oil can easily be melted in the microwave in 30 seconds.

Makes six to eight muffins

2 eggs
1 ripe banana
2 tbsp cold-pressed coconut oil, melted
2 oz / 55 g oat flour
1¼ oz / 35 g rolled oats
1 tbsp psyllium husk
1 tsp baking powder
1 tsp ground cardamom
pinch salt
1¾ oz / 50 g raspberries

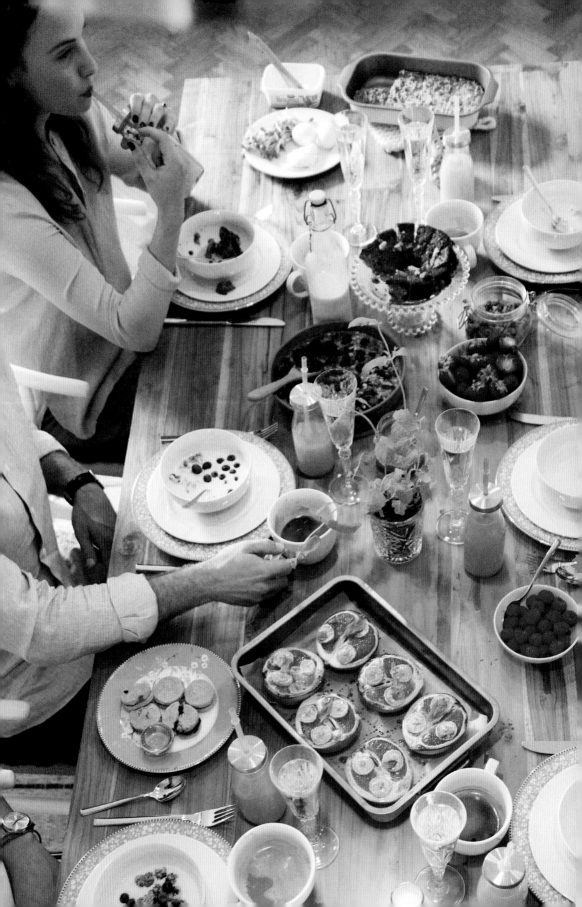

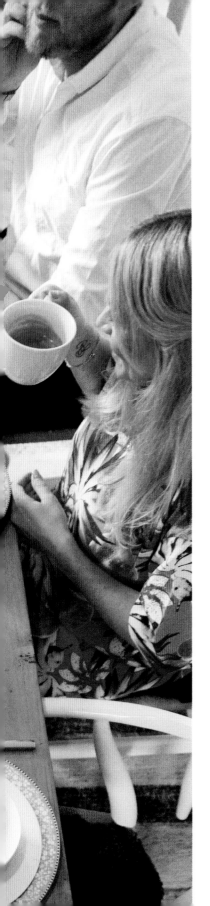

Weekend brunch for friends

ONE WAY OF BRIGHTENING UP your morning is to eat breakfast in company—everyone appreciates a good brunch.

It's great to meet up in town, but I prefer to host brunch in my own kitchen when we can sit, nibble, and chat for several hours. I meet friends for brunch regularly, whatever the time of day. It is a lovely way to bring people together, and everyone gets to decide which of their favorite dishes to bring along.

The recipes in this chapter take a little more time and are ideally prepared jointly. Some people prefer something a bit more filling for brunch but, as the breakfast lover I am, I like to have freshly-baked bread, tasty accompaniments, juice, and something sweet. And the best thing is—there is something for everyone!

BANANA LOAF

Makes one loaf

3 ripe bananas

6–8 fresh dates, pitted

4 eggs

4½ oz / 125 g hazelnut flour

2½ oz / 70 g shredded coconut

3 tbsp cold-pressed coconut oil, melted

2 tsp baking powder

1 tsp vanilla powder

pinch salt

This is one of my favorite recipes. If I have bananas in the house that are almost too ripe, I make a banana loaf. The bananas and dates in the mixture mean no other sweeteners are needed, and the loaf is lovely and soft but with a crisp crust.

METHOD:

Heat the oven to 360 °F / 180 °C. Use a stick blender to blend the banana and dates into a sticky mixture. Add the other ingredients. Grease a bread or cake tin with coconut oil and pour in the mixture. Bake in the middle of the oven for 45–50 minutes. Allow to cool before serving.

Eat as it is, or with jam, chocolate-hazelnut spread, or nut butter (see recipes on page 128).

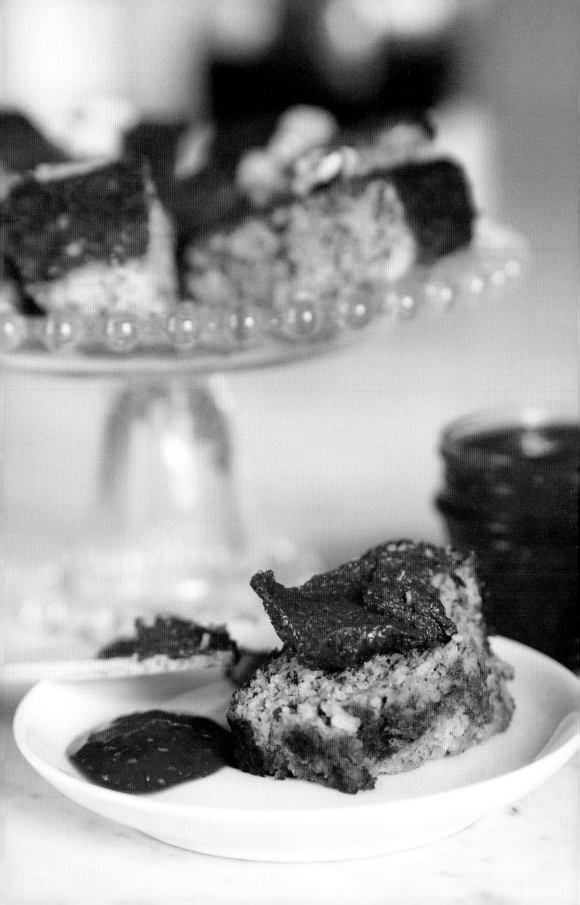

CHOCOLATE-HAZELNUT SPREAD

Makes one big jar

9 oz / 260 g hazelnuts
1½ oz / 40 g raw cacao powder
⅓ cup / 75 ml hazelnut milk or nut milk of your choice
1 tbsp cold-pressed coconut oil, melted
2 tsp vanilla powder
1½ tsp stevia powder
salt

I still remember when I was given chocolate-hazelnut spread for the first time as a child. I've loved it ever since and nowadays I like to make a version of my own. Chocolate-hazelnut spread is equally good spread on freshly baked bread as it is served with banana pancakes or accompanying fresh fruit as a dessert. This recipe makes a crunchy, nutty version!

METHOD:
Heat the oven to 390 °F / 200 °C. Spread out the hazelnuts on a baking tray covered with parchment paper and roast in the middle of the oven for 10–15 minutes. Allow the nuts to cool a little and rub off the skin with your hands.

Grind the nuts into hazelnut butter in a food processor. The nuts will initially turn into a powder but after a while they will release their oil and the mixture will become creamier. Be patient, it will work out eventually.

Add the other ingredients, and taste to ensure you get a good balance between sweetness and saltiness.

NUT BUTTER

Makes one small jar

generous ¾ cup / 200 ml nuts, e.g. almonds, hazelnuts, or peanuts
pinch sea salt flakes

METHOD:
Heat the oven to 390 °F / 200 °C. Spread out the nuts on a baking tray covered with parchment paper and toast in the middle of the oven for 12 minutes until golden brown. Then, pulse them in a food processor with a pinch of sea salt flakes. You'll need to process in stages.

Initially the nuts will become a dry powder, and then, eventually, a paste. Pause the food processor a few times so that it does not overheat and scrape the paste down from the sides of the container. Soon the almonds or nuts will release their oil and then you simply continue to blend until you have a creamy butter. Taste and add more salt if necessary.

Store the nut butter in a glass jar in the fridge, where it will keep for four or five days.

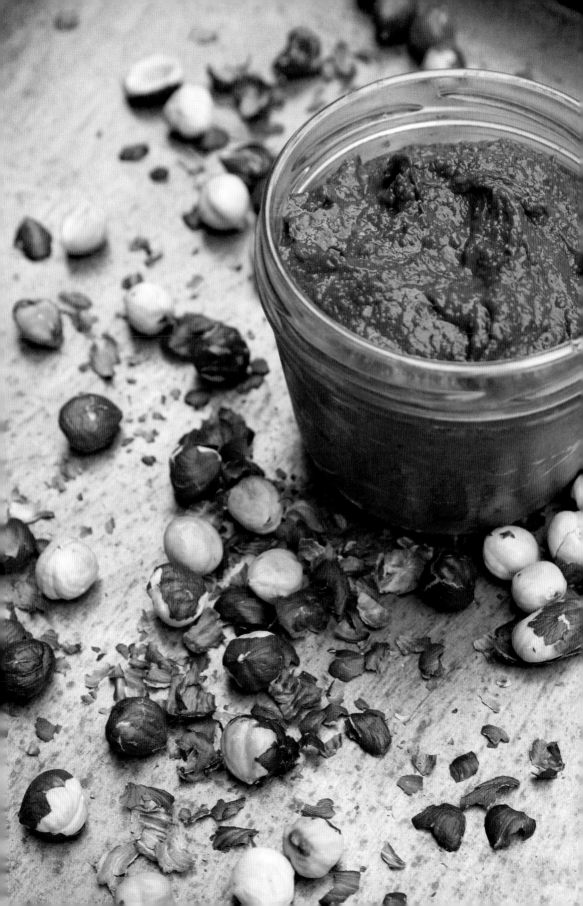

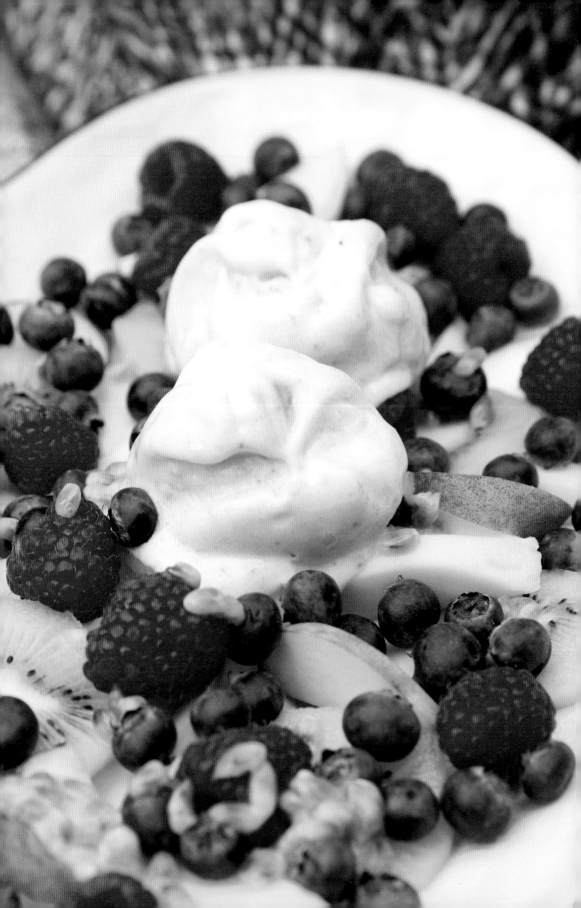

FRUIT SALAD WITH BANANA ICE CREAM

This fruit salad with banana ice cream is almost too good to count as a breakfast, but it is exactly the sort of dish that belongs in a brunch! I have also served it as a healthy dessert, and the ice cream goes down very well with both adults and children.

METHOD:

Start with the banana ice cream. Peel and slice the bananas and put them in a plastic bag in the freezer for at least four hours. Take them out a couple of minutes before you want to serve the ice cream and allow them to defrost just a little before adding the vanilla powder and blending with a stick blender to a smooth, ice cream-like consistency. Use really ripe bananas—they are sweet and delicious.

Serve the ice cream with sliced fruit and fresh berries.

Tip

This is such a simple recipe, and can be varied in a multitude of ways. Try adding cacao for a sweet banana and chocolate ice cream, or mango or frozen berries for a fruitier result. A stick blender works best here—in an ordinary blender, the bananas will often stick in the blades.

Makes two portions

Banana ice cream:
3 ripe bananas
½ tsp vanilla powder

Fruit salad:
1 peach
1 kiwi
1 ripe mango
1 passion fruit
2 oz / 60 g fresh
  blueberries
1¾ oz / 50 g fresh
  raspberries

CHIA JAM

Makes one small jar

2 tbsp chia seeds

⅔ cup / 150 ml water

7 oz / 200 g fruit and
berries of your choice,
e.g. peach, raspberries,
blueberries, apples,
figs

pinch vanilla powder

1 tbsp freshly-squeezed
lemon juice

approx. 1 tsp honey,
depending on the
sweetness of the fruit/
berries

Homemade jam is tastier and healthier than jam bought from a store.
You can also flavor it exactly as you want and use combinations of
different fruits and berries. Do some experimenting to find out what
you like best.

METHOD:

Mix the chia seeds and the water. Stir until there are no dry seeds on
the surface and allow to stand for five minutes. Using a stick blender,
blend the fruit and berries, then add the chia mixture and continue to
blend. Flavor with vanilla powder, lemon, and honey to taste, if liked.
Put the jam in the fridge for a few minutes to allow it to settle. It will
keep in the fridge for three or four days.

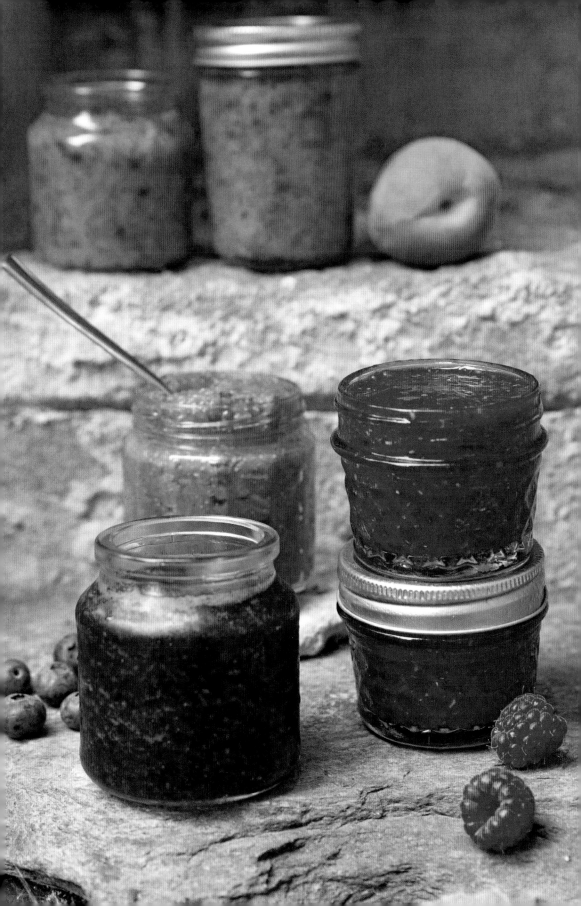

BUCKWHEAT WAFFLES WITH CHIA JAM

Makes four portions

generous ¾ cup /
200 ml oat milk
11 oz / 300 g buckwheat
  flour
2 tsp baking powder
2 eggs
generous ¾ cup /
  200 ml ice-cold water,
  ideally carbonated
1 tsp salt
pinch vanilla powder

For cooking:
cold-pressed coconut oil

What would a brunch be without waffles? These crispy waffles are made from buckwheat flour and they are simply delicious with chia jam and some whipped coconut cream.

METHOD:

Mix the oat milk with the buckwheat flour and baking powder. Add the eggs one at a time; pour in the cold water, salt, and vanilla powder; and whisk into a smooth batter. Carbonated water makes fluffier waffles. Cook in a waffle iron using the coconut oil and serve hot and crispy along with the chia jam from page 132.

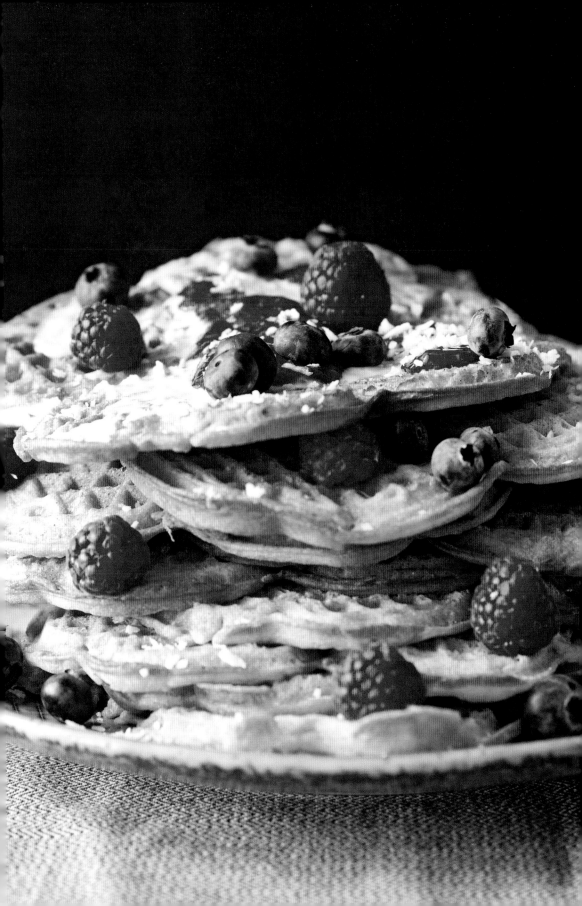

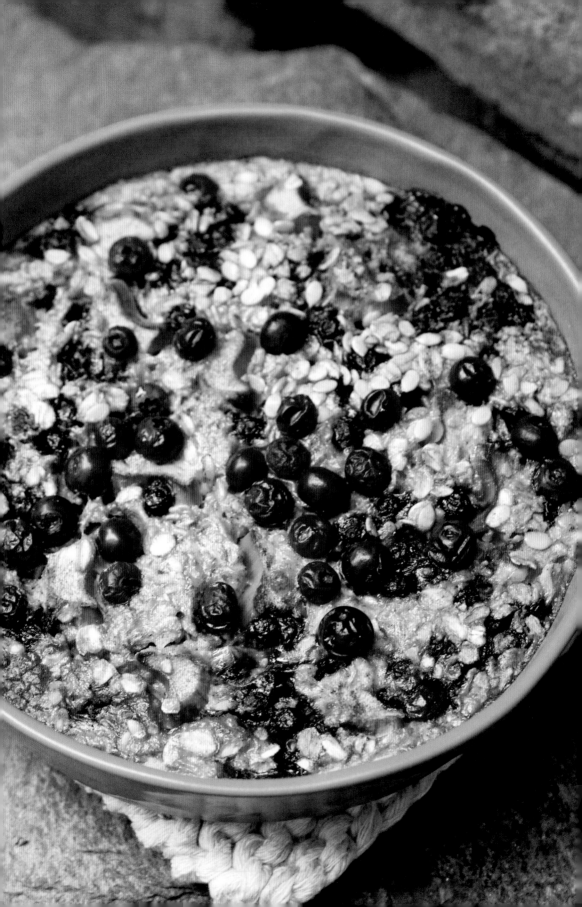

BAKED OATS WITH BLUEBERRIES AND RHUBARB

A scrumptious mixture of oat porridge and berry pie. Baking in a flan tin gives a much more luxurious feeling, and it is perfect for a weekend breakfast or brunch with friends.

METHOD:

Heat the oven to 360 °F / 180 °C. Grease a baking tin (approx. 9 in. / 23 cm in diameter) with the coconut oil. Mix all the dry ingredients together and pour into the tin. Whisk the eggs and almond milk and pour them over the mixture in the tin. Top with the blueberries, sliced rhubarb, seeds of your choice (I usually use sunflower and pumpkin seeds), and some honey.

Bake in the center of the oven for 30–35 minutes until the bake is a lovely golden brown. Serve with cold almond milk.

Makes four to six portions

2 tsp cold-pressed coconut oil
5 oz / 140 g rolled oats
1 tsp baking powder
1 tsp vanilla powder
2 tsp ground cinnamon
1 tsp sea salt flakes
3 eggs
1²⁄₃ cups / 400 ml almond milk
6½ oz / 180 g blueberries
4 oz / 120 g rhubarb, sliced
seeds of your choice
1 tbsp honey

To serve:
almond milk

FRUIT PANCAKE

Makes two portions

1 egg
1 egg white
7 tbsp / 100 ml almond
  milk
2 oz / 55 g almond flour
1 tsp honey
1 tsp cold-pressed
  coconut oil, melted
  + 1 tsp for frying
pinch vanilla powder
small pinch salt
peach, blueberries, and
  strawberries (2 oz /
  60 g in total)
runny honey to serve

A luxurious fruit pancake that you bake in the oven with fresh fruit and fresh berries.

METHOD:

Heat the oven to 390 °F / 200 °C. Whisk all the ingredients apart from the fruit until you have a fluffy batter. Pour the batter into a small frying pan greased with a little coconut oil, and place in the oven for two to three minutes until set. Slice the peach and the strawberries. Remove the frying pan, top with the fruit and berries, and put back into the oven for eight to ten minutes until the pancake is golden brown.

Drizzle over the honey and serve immediately.

Tip

If there are more than two of you, double the quantities, and make the pancake in a bigger frying pan.

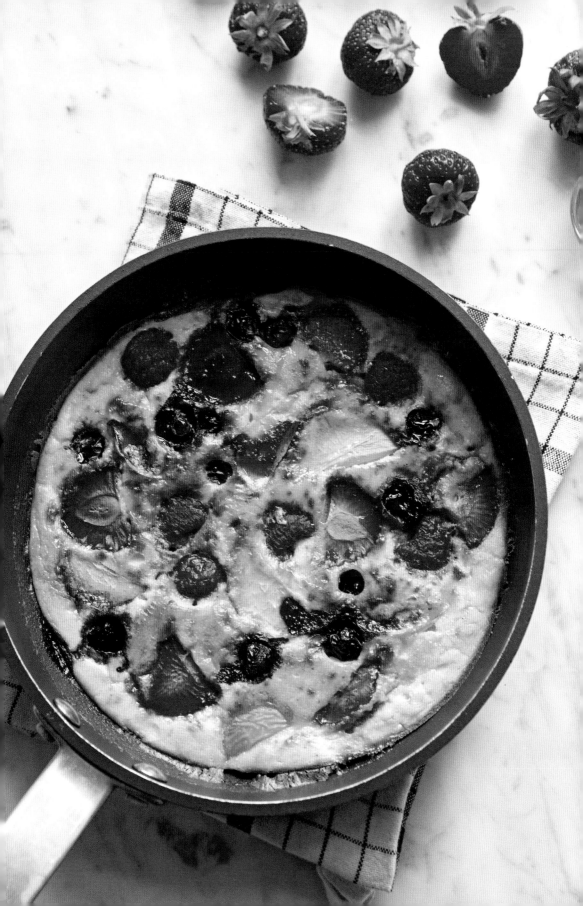

PEAR, KIWI, AND PINEAPPLE JUICE

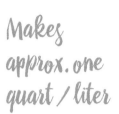

Makes approx. one quart / liter

6 kiwifruit
5 pears
1 pineapple

It always feels luxurious to be able to serve freshly-squeezed juice in small bottles. This green juice is both sweet and sour and will give your table a wonderful splash of color.

METHOD:
Peel the kiwifruit and the pineapple and slice the pears into small pieces (these do not need to be peeled). Juice everything in a juice extractor, slow juicer, or whatever you prefer to use. Serve in small bottles or in glasses with ice.

Tip

If you do not have a juice extractor, you can make the juice just as easily in a blender. Core the pears, peel the kiwifruit and the pineapple, and cut the fruit into small pieces. Blend the fruit with a little water and strain the resulting liquid using a strainer or a nut milk bag.

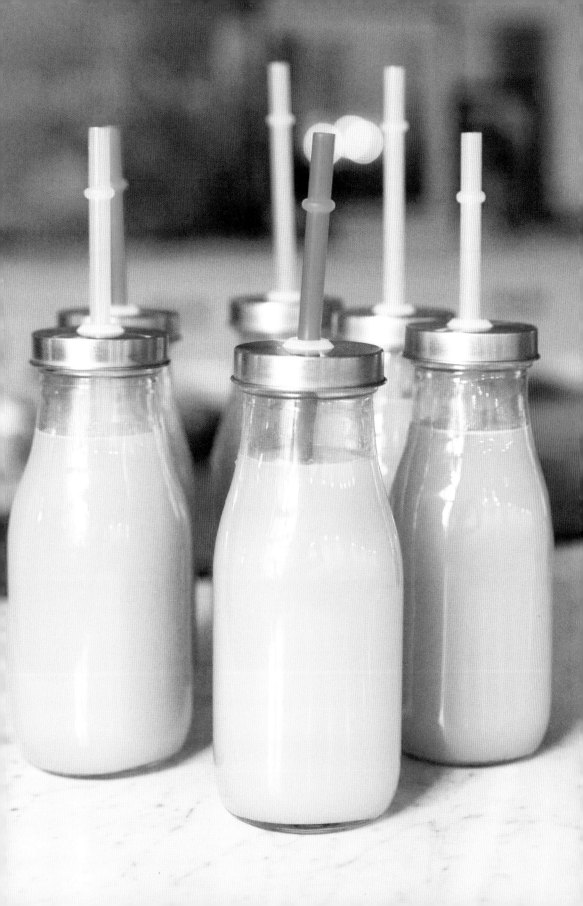

GRAPEFRUIT AU GRATIN

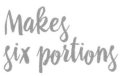

Makes six portions

3 grapefruit
2 bananas
1 tbsp honey
sprig mint for
  decoration

This is a fun breakfast trend that I picked up in New York. The acidity of the grapefruit and sweetness of the banana and honey are a perfect match. It is as delicious to eat as it is lovely to look at.

METHOD:

Heat the oven to 360 °F / 180 °C. Halve the grapefruit and place it on a baking tray covered with parchment paper. Place some sliced banana on the grapefruit and drizzle with honey. Bake in the middle of the oven for 10–12 minutes until the banana starts to turn a nice golden-brown color.

Serve with fresh mint and eat with a knife and fork.

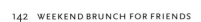

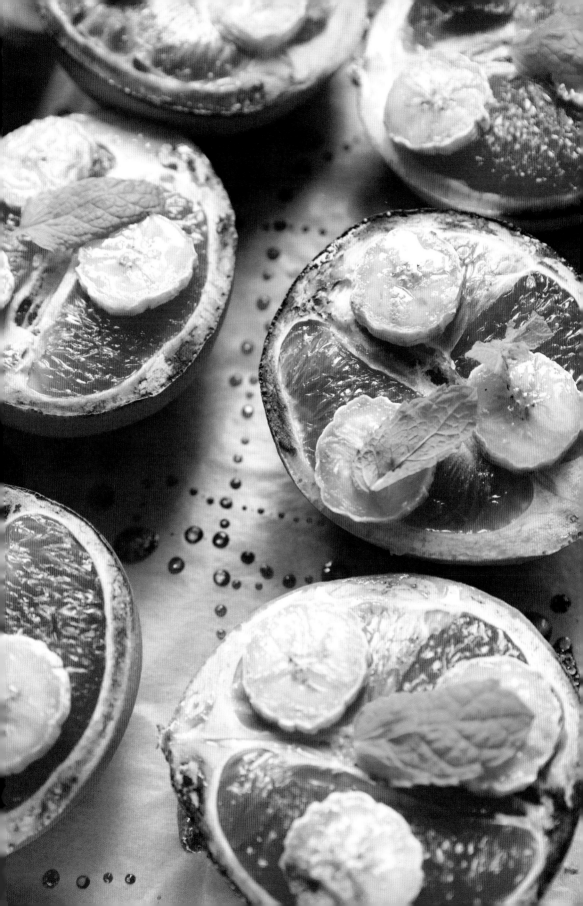

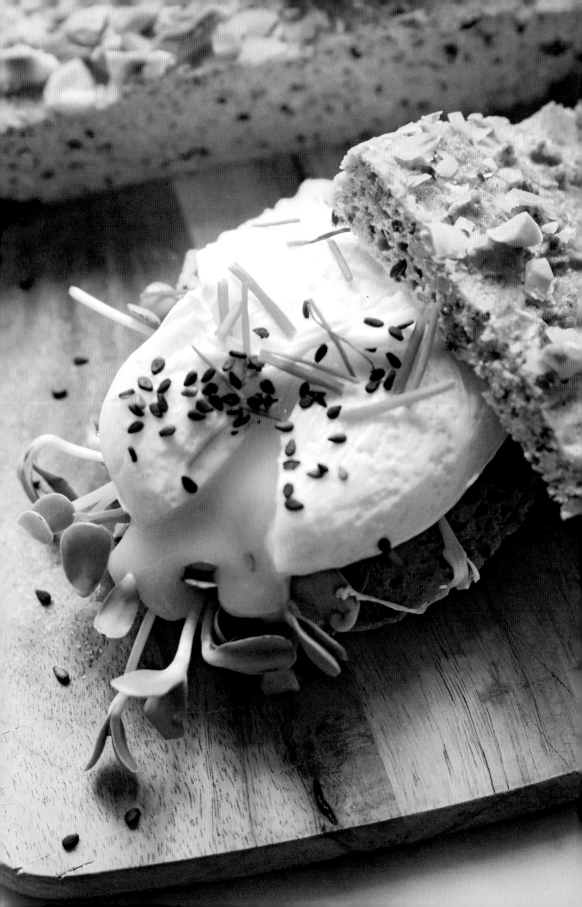

CARROT BREAD

A fluffy, moist almond and carrot bread—easy to bake and popular with the whole family. When serving it for brunch, I like to accompany it with poached egg and some greens, as in the picture.

METHOD:
Heat the oven to 360 °F / 180 °C. Cut the carrots into small pieces and blend in a food processor. Mix in the almond milk and eggs and blend again. Mix all the dry ingredients together in a bowl and blend together with the other ingredients in the food processor.

Grease a baking pan, bread pan, or spring-form tin with coconut oil and pour in the mixture. Top with chopped almonds and bake in the center of the oven for about 30 minutes until the bread is golden brown.

Makes one loaf

2 carrots, peeled
generous ¾ cup /
  200 ml unsweetened
  almond milk
2 eggs
5 oz / 140 g almond flour
4 oz / 115 g buckwheat
  flour
2 tbsp psyllium husk
2 tbsp cold-pressed
  coconut oil, melted
3 tsp baking powder
3½ tbsp / 50 ml crushed
  flaxseeds
salt
coconut oil for greasing

Topping:
blanched, chopped
  almonds

MANGO LASSI BOWL

Makes six to eight portions

1 quart / 1 liter oat yogurt, soy yogurt, or yogurt of your choice
4 frozen bananas
10 oz / 280 g frozen mango

I serve this creamy mango lassi with my granola instead of yogurt (see granola recipe on page 92). Using oat yogurt as a base gives it the perfect tanginess.

METHOD:

Allow the mango and banana to defrost for a few minutes at room temperature. Blend together with the oat yogurt into a creamy mango lassi. You may want to add more water depending on the desired consistency.

Did you know?

Oat yogurt is a dairy-free yogurt based on oat drink. It is suitable for sensitive stomachs, rich in oat fiber, and a good base for creamy smoothies. You can also use soy yogurt or ordinary yogurt to make your lassi.

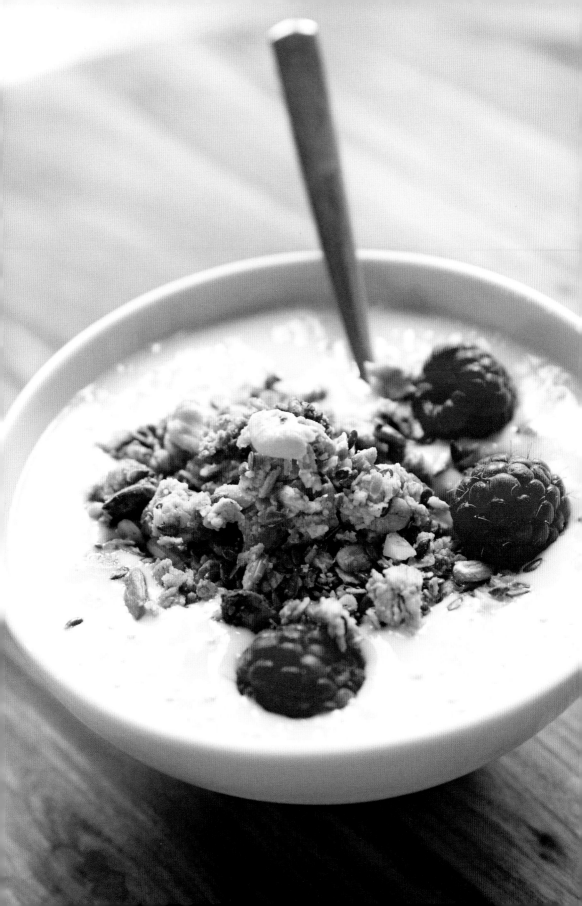

EGGS IN AVOCADO AU GRATIN

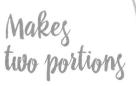

Makes two portions

1 avocado
2 small eggs
salt and pepper

This is an interesting and rather novel way to eat eggs. The avocado retains both its texture and its taste while in the oven and goes perfectly with the eggs. Healthy, tasty, and really easy to make.

METHOD:
Heat the oven to 390 °F / 200 °C. Halve and pit a ripe avocado. Scoop enough flesh out of the avocado to allow room for an egg. Crack an egg into each avocado half and season with salt and pepper. Bake in the oven for 10 minutes until the yolk has just set.

Tip

This is particularly tasty if you sprinkle some grated parmesan and chili powder over the avocado before you put it in the oven so that it is crispy on top.

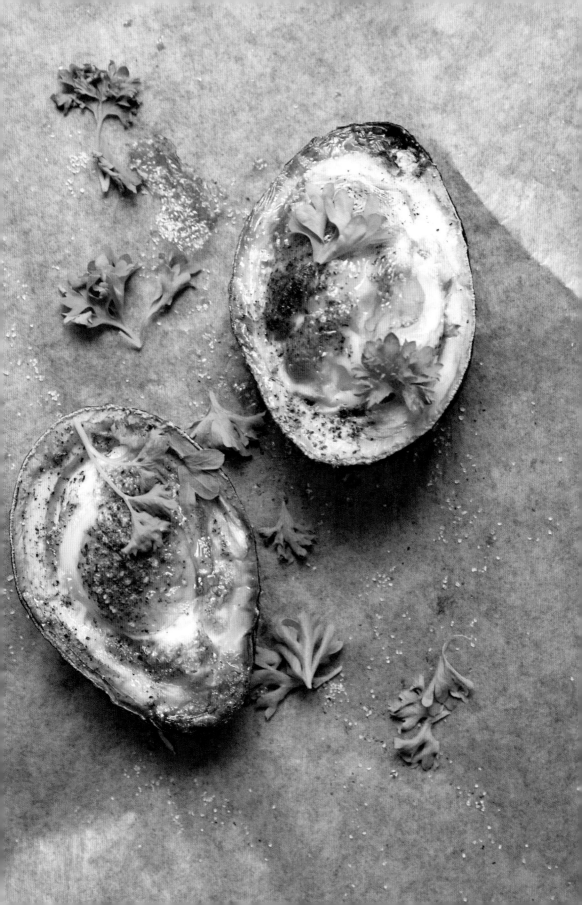

INDEX

Thank you!

To Marcus—my love, my best friend, and my biggest supporter. To my family for believing in me come what may, and for giving me the confidence to try new things. To Iman and Johan, for allowing us to photograph inside your amazing apartment. To Maria and family, for letting us have use of your little piece of heaven in the archipelago. Last but not least, thanks to Norstedts and in especially Michaéla, Åsa, Pernilla, and Charlotte for making this book more beautiful than I had dared to imagine. Thank you too to my faithful readers, who have made all of this possible—this book is for you.

Abbreviations and Quantities

1 oz = 1 ounce = 28 grams
1 lb = 1 pound = 16 ounces
1 cup = approx. 5–8 ounces* (see below)
1 cup = 8 fluid ounces = 250 milliliters (liquids)
2 cups = 1 pint (liquids) = 500 milliliters (liquids)
8 pints = 4 quarts = 1 gallon (liquids)
1 g = 1 gram = 1/1000 kilogram = 5 ml (liquids)
1 kg = 1 kilogram = 1000 grams = 2¼ lb
1 l = 1 liter = 1000 milliliters (ml) = 1 quart
125 milliliters (ml) = approx. 8 tablespoons = ½ cup
1 tbsp = 1 level tablespoon = 15–20 g* (depending on density) = 15 milliliters (liquids)
1 tsp = 1 level teaspoon = 3–5 g * (depending on density) = 5 ml (liquids)

*The weight of dry ingredients varies significantly depending on the density factor, e.g. 1 cup of flour weighs less than 1 cup of butter. Quantities in ingredients have been rounded up or down for convenience, where appropriate. Metric conversions may therefore not correspond exactly. It is important to use either American or metric measurements within a recipe.

First published by Norstedts, Sweden, in 2016
Published by agreement with Norstedts Agency
En god morgon – Härliga frukostar för en bra start
ISBN of the original edition: 978-91-1-307095-7

Text © Anja Forsnor
Photographs/Illustrations © Charlotte Gawell
Design: Pernilla Qvist
Editor: Åsa Karsberg

© for the English edition: h.f. ullmann publishing GmbH
Translation from Swedish: Edwina Simpson in association with First Edition Translations Ltd, Cambridge, UK

Overall responsibility of production: h.f. ullmann publishing GmbH, Potsdam, Germany

Printed in Slovenia, 2017

ISBN 978-3-8480-1115-5

10 9 8 7 6 5 4 3 2 1
X IX VIII VII VI V IV III II I

www.ullmannmedien.com
info@ullmannmedien.com
facebook.com/ullmannmedien
twitter.com/ullmann_int

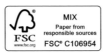

FSC
MIX
Paper from responsible sources
www.fsc.org   FSC® C106954